What Others Are Saying...

"Cathi is genuinely concerned about the health and wellness of others and has a gift to heal what ails a body. I am so thankful that I know her and will continue to seek her guidance and healing. I am also firm believer in fate; I was meant to meet Cathi and she was meant to "fix" me."

—Debbie McCrossan
Certified Personal Trainer (CPT) and
licensed provider of the Tupler Technique

"Our readers love Cathi Stack's column in our Sunday lifestyle pages. Her topics are always cutting edge and her information thoroughly researched and easy to understand. I consider her words to be a community service to our readers."

—Michele DeLuca
Features Editor, Niagara Gazette

"This book has a wealth of information that can have you feeling better than you ever thought you could. Cathi has provided an invaluable resource for those who are living with chronic disease or need assistance in healing. I have experienced her healing abilities personally and have seen what she has done for others. This is gift to all who read it."

—Patricia Chapin
RT(T) Certified in Nutritional and Lifestyle Oncology

Free Yourself from a

CONSTIPATED

Life

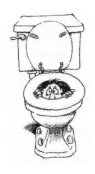

CATHERINE STACK, N.D., C.N.M.

Free Yourself from a CONSTIPATED Life
Catherine Stack, N.D., C.N.M.

ISBN: 978-0-6157894-6-0

This book is for educational purposes only. It is not a substitution for medical advice. Please consult your personal health care providers for your individual health concerns. Neither Catherine Stack nor Journey II Health have any responsibility for any adverse effects arising directly or indirectly as a result of the information provided in this book. Trademark names may be used throughout this book. Rather than put a trademark symbol after every occurrence of a trademark name, we used names in an editorial fashion only, and to the benefit of the trademark owner, with no intention of infringement of the trademark.

First Printing 2013

Cover Design by Tracy Bloom (etbloomer@gmail.com)
Book Layout and Editing by Lindsey Wiler
(lindseywiler@gmail.com)

This book is dedicated to all the constipated individuals who suffer silently and have yet to find help,

...until now.

Contents

*PART TWO: CONSTIPATION IN OTHER
AREAS OF YOUR LIFE*

Acknowledgements

F irst and foremost, I'd like to thank all my patients who have taught me so much about the mind body connection. Your experiences teach me everyday and there is no textbook that could teach all that you have shared. A special thanks to Anne, as she takes us the farthest with her story: death, beyond, and back. You are truly a gift in my life and your sweetness needs to stay here on earth for a good long while.

To Patrick, my ever-supportive husband, who was used to having me around much more than I am now. Most husbands would not have tolerated my whimsical ideas and career changes as you have. I am so fortunate to have had the constant support so that I may spread my wings and fly. The love continues to grow deep and I am forever grateful.

To my coworkers at Journey II Health—JeriAnn Delmonte, Marie Maio and Lindsey Wiler, my "Journey Queens". Without your support and creativity I would not have time or the desire for any other projects. Finishing this book would not be possible without the editing, formatting and re-editing that Lindsey has endured. I know there were many "after" hours spent on this tedious process. I am grateful for all your diversity and commitment to make Journey II Health what it is and what it is evolving to become.

To all my friends and coworkers on the Millard

Fillmore Suburban Labor Wing, you keep me loving my job as a midwife. You make me laugh, keep my adrenalin pumping and most of all, nurture my soul. A position I could never leave easily.

To my loving and supportive sister Patti, you help to keep me so connected on the happenings around the family when my life is so busy. You have a magical way of balancing what's most important in life and always take the time to connect and make sure all is well. You are a great cancer coach—you have so much to offer.

To Marie Coyle, my mom, thanks for your editing help and so much more. I can't help but laugh when I think back to the girl who just wanted out of high school and still couldn't spell...who would have thought? Thank you for believing in me and putting many of my recommendations into motion. Having you around for a long, long time is a blessing. Having parents who told me I could do anything from a very early age—priceless! (Parents, please tell your children from a very early age that they can do or be anything they want. This penetrates to a cellular level, which will positively impact the lives of your children.)

To my children, Josh and Sam, you have made motherhood a very rewarding experience for which I have many amazing memories to cherish. I hope you both have the opportunity to experience the happiness and joy of having such great children. Sam, thank you for the amazing cover! Only in my dreams could my abs look so good. You are beautiful.

To Tracy Bloom, whose artistic eye and ability never cease to amaze me. Thank you for sharing your gift of style and design for the cover of one of my favorite projects to date.

"Nobody can go back and start a new beginning, but anyone can start today and create a new ending."

—Maria Robinson

How To Use This Book

As you read, you will find yourself relating to many of the personal stories and scenarios in this book. I have added blank pages to the end of this book so that you may take notes, jot down mentioned remedies, or highlight page numbers you'd like to go back and read. There is so much information in this book and one of the most difficult tasks was trying to organize it.

Don't lend this book out! I have done this with some of my most beloved books and have yet to get them back. There is too much good advice given here and you will want to reference it often. I hope it serves you well.

Introduction

We are all in one way, shape or form, constipated. It may be in our job, our relationships, or literally in our bowel. When we are not constipated, life flows as effortless as a river going downhill. Doors open up, opportunities present themselves, and life is easy.

This book is a summary of the work I do in and out of every week. It is an accumulation of my experience in the healing arts for twenty-six plus years. My career has taken me along a path that began as a young, inexperienced night nurse, to a teacher, a midwife, colon therapist, and a doctor of naturopathy. And so evolves an interesting but fulfilling life I could have never predicted. One thing I know for sure is that my life purpose is to continue on this healing path in whatever form it has in store for me.

Of all the degrees and education I have received, it is my colon hydrotherapy training that has been the most rewarding. Constipated individuals are everywhere. They can't think, they are uncomfortable, miserable, and oh are they toxic! They will ultimately suffer from other related ailments if their constipation is not resolved. Constipation is today's version of a plague that may very well expedite our exit from this planet.

Show someone how to fix their issue of constipation and they are not likely to ever let themselves slip back into the uncomfortable abyss. Unfortunately, many get little help from their doctors and specialists. Eventually the supplements and medications that once worked are no longer providing benefit and leaving them back to the drawing board.

My experience with people is life-long. At 15 years of age I had the opportunity to volunteer at my local hospital in the emergency department. It is an experience I value to this day and will never forget. I was probably better equipped to save someone's life during that time than when I was fresh out of nursing school and even now. I have worked with people in a healing capacity my entire life and am grateful for the way it has enriched and shaped my life. Yes, I have the degrees, but it is in my human contact where I have found the most value when it comes to my education.

What has kept me motivated to finish this book is that no matter where I go, I will inevitably meet someone who is uncomfortable with constipation. It sadly affects the travel or conference that they had been looking forward to, and relief from their constipation becomes a distracting obsession. While writing this book, I attended a workshop given by a popular publishing company. At the beginning of this conference, I had the pleasure of meeting a wonderful woman I'll call Karen. Karen was in her late fifties and more excited about writing her book and a possible move in order to change the whole direction of her life. She was lovely and vibrant. By day two of the conference, she was losing the vibrancy and actually seemed a bit distracted. I asked if everything was OK, thinking she might not be sleeping well. She confided in me that whenever she travels, she becomes constipated and was becoming very uncomfortable. What a shame! She was now very distracted and was losing her focus on why she was here, but I knew this was my sign—I was here for a reason.

Because I myself rarely suffer from constipation, I was not in the habit of bringing my "tools" with me. I now travel with a small supply of supplements that will usually relieve the constipated traveler.

I have a library full of books on health and nutrition. Not one of them focuses on constipation. Some don't even mention it. A poor state of affairs in the digestive tract will fast track the downfall of your health—period. Many seemingly unrelated symptoms would be eliminated if one would just focus on the health of their colon.

A common question I get during a colon hydrotherapy session (colonic) is, "What made you want to do this?" Most individuals think I must be crazy and I myself would have asked the same question. If you had told me years ago that I would be helping to deliver people from their poop, as well as delivering babies, I would have looked at you as if you had lost your mind. Simply stated, when I hand you that beautiful baby, you have your work cut out for you for the next 18 years or more. When I deliver you from your constipation, you will soon know what it is like to feel fabulous.

I am not trying to downplay the absolute beauty of birth, but for the purpose of this book, we need to focus our attention on pooping well. Relieving you from a constipated colon is my objective. Relieving you from a constipated life will only bring you freedom and joy in whatever it is you are on this planet for. I will give you all my tried and true remedies that will help, even if you decide colon hydrotherapy is not for you. (Described in detail in Chapter 6). It is important to realize that you may also be constipated in other areas, as most constipated individuals are. Whether it is your health, thoughts, relationships or spiritual beliefs, this book will hopefully guide you in resolving other areas of constipation in your life.

There is no pill, quick fix or fad diet that will add years to your precious life. Falling for these options will likely shave precious years off your life or at the very least, diminish the productive quality. We were born with the free will to live and eat as we choose. What I don't understand is why people choose to live physically handicapped with illness, obesity and inflammation when they don't have to.

The saddest scenario in modern medicine is that we do not see the direct connection between what we put in our mouths and our state of health. It is almost too easy, and yet ultimately ignored!

Who you become over the next few years will depend on the large majority of what foods you put in your mouth from this day forward. Depending on your age and current state of health, you may actually feel ten years younger in a very short period of time. What you now have in your hands are all the tools that I use on a daily basis with my patients. It is my mission to heal beyond the walls of my practice and to infiltrate the local community and beyond.

MY GOAL IS TO "MOVE" YOU, at least twice daily. If you lose a few pounds, achieve better health, feel optimistic and vibrant, I have done my job.

Removing the crap in your colon (and your life)

opens the space for new and better things. Clean up your internal environment and you'll be surprised how your external environment improves as well.

The supplements I use for my patients are described in detail and readily available to you via Internet, our website (www.journeyiihealth.com) or in natural health stores in your area.

I have included interesting stories and perspectives from my patients. Most of them are told in their own words and share a story that so many of you will understand and relate to. Some have let me use their names; others have requested I change them. Anne's story is probably the driving force behind this book. There are more like her out there. You will be touched by her story and it may save a few lives.

Maybe this book will become one of your favorite bathroom reads. So for the constipated individual, you will have plenty of reading time. My intention is that as your digestive health improves (because you've read this book)—you won't need to sit there very long.

Remember this: You are always your own best doctor as you take a proactive approach to your health and listen to your intuition. I am very excited for you as you begin your quest for better health, and I look forward to hearing your success stories. You can let me know at journeyiihealth@gmail.com.

Be well and enjoy the journey!

—Cathi

PART ONE

LITERALLY CONSTIPATED

A ccording to the National Digestive Diseases Information Clearinghouse (NDDIC) from 2000-2004, over 63 million people suffer from chronic constipation in the United States alone. 6.3 million have been seen for constipation in the ambulatory setting, while 700,000 have been hospitalized. Approximately 5.3 million prescriptions are written each year for this problem alone. Sadly, very few resolve the issue.

Constipation is a pandemic throughout the world in developed and industrialized countries. It does not discriminate between men, women, children, race or religion. Even those who drink plenty of water and eat a clean, healthy diet are not immune.

This section provides a collection of constipated scenarios and most of you will find yourselves somewhere in the pages ahead. A "one size fits all" remedy does not exist when it comes to treating constipation. I wish it could be that simple.

I have spent a large portion of the past decade helping chronically constipated individuals resolve issues that may have even plagued them during childhood. It is through these experiences that I bring you a variety of helpful tips, even for the most challenging individuals. There is hope, there is help.

Chapter 1

Anatomy of the CONSTIPATED Individual

B efore we move on, it would be best to give you a brief and simple anatomy lesson about the colon and its function. The colon is approximately five feet in length, and for those who haven't over-distended things, about 2.5 inches in diameter. (Most of us have over-distended things). It is a muscular organ. The main function of the colon is to reabsorb liquid, taking your waste from a very liquid state to a solid state. The longer the waste remains in the colon, the harder and denser it becomes. This reduces you to a few bunny pellets here and there while things begin to become uncomfortably distended.

There are many constipated individuals who are not uncomfortable. This is because when things happen gradually over long periods of time, the body may not notice. Other functions of the colon include: fermentation of food by-products with the help of bacteria, excretion of poisonous waste, storage of waste products until time of elimination, and excretion of toxic waste. (We hope).

The majority of nutrient absorption takes place in the small intestine, but up to 15 percent takes place in the first half of the large intestine. Vitamins that depend on a clean colon are A, D, K and E.

Bacteria in the Colon

Within the colon, huge populations of a variety of bacteria go to work in order to break down waste. The stomach and small intestine have a much smaller population of bacteria when compared to the colon. Intestinal flora accounts for 2-5 pounds of our total body weight and has up to 2000 different species.

There are basically two major categories of bacteria within the colon, the good guys and the bad guys. In a healthy colon, the good bacteria should account for 85 percent of the population, leaving the 15 percent to the bad guys. What most individuals don't realize is that 80 percent of your immune system lies within your gastrointestinal tract.

Unfortunately, the Standard American Diet (SAD) has caused many individuals to harbor more unfriendly bacteria than beneficial. This fragile state of health predisposes the individual to illness, especially food related, far easier than someone with a healthy balance. Add to that the overuse or misuse of antibiotics, which also destroy the healthy bacteria, and you become an easy target for intestinal trouble.

Friendly bacteria within the colon are very important to overall health. It is very important to replace the healthy bacteria with a quality probiotic supplement following any antibiotic treatment.

Many individuals walk around with the diagnosis of Irritable Bowel Syndrome (IBS) and I am surprised at how many individuals are "cured" after initiating the use of some high quality probiotics and dietary changes.

Candida

Candida (yeast) is a common complication of a colon and digestive system gone wrong, due to the lack of healthy bacteria needed for protection. A significant number of people suffer from systemic Candida, or more commonly, yeast.

Candida has a chameleon-like ability to change from non-invasive, sugar-fermenting yeast to a fungal form that has long root-like structures that can penetrate the intestinal mucosa. This condition is commonly referred to as Leaky Gut Syndrome, which is responsible for releasing toxins into the blood stream. This, in turn, leads to a wide range of problems from bloating, constipation and gas, food sensitivities, allergies, skin rashes, Chronic Fatigue Syndrome and eventually autoimmune disease.

Slow wound healing is also common with Candida overgrowth. When people take antibiotics to cure infection or illness, they fail to recognize that the good, health-protecting bacteria are also destroyed, leaving yeast (Candida) to flourish and take over. It is the beneficial bacteria that will keep Candida at bay in a healthy body. The overuse of antibiotics is partially responsible for the large numbers of people who suffer from systemic Candida. Even antibiotic residues in commercial meat contribute to setting the stage for overgrowth. Other common medications that contribute to yeast overgrowth are birth control pills and steroids.

Many physicians are not familiar with treating Candida overgrowth, as the symptoms are usually nonspecific and vague. Irritable Bowel Syndrome is a common label. In women, the diagnosis of a yeast infection is simple to make and easy to treat. Those who suffer from an occasional vaginal yeast infection are likely loaded in the gut and should consider systemic treatment. The problem with using with topical and oral preparations such as Monistat and Diflucan is that it will potentially lead to resistant Candida issues. These medications work well initially, but because the underlying cause is rarely addressed, results are usually temporary and overgrowth will most likely strike again. If diet and supplementation are not addressed, the medicinal action is only likely to suppress, not eradicate, the problem.

Sugar, which is Candida's favorite food, along with a diet full of refined carbohydrates (breads, crackers, etc.), makes the battle almost impossible to win. A strict Candida diet must be followed for at least two months or more. This diet eliminates most dairy, all sugar, most fruits, alcohol, and bread products. This leaves you with what nature intended you to eat anyway. Fish, vegetables, meat, poultry, lots of pure water, herbal teas (especially Pau d'Arco) and some whole grains such as quinoa and rice would have you feeling spectacular in a very short period of time. Emphasis should be placed on foods known to have anti-fungal properties such as garlic, onions, broccoli, cabbage, kale, collards, Brussels sprouts, olive and flax oils, cinnamon and cloves.

The symptoms of getting rid of systemic yeast can feel almost flu-like for a few days, but the downside is usually short-lived. The sugar cravings may be pretty intense as well—the yeast want to be fed. Do you really want to feed the bad guys? Don't give in! Diet modifications, as discussed above, are going to make or break your success when it comes to eradicating yeast. Nutritional supplements such as probiotics (healthy bacteria), colloidal silver, vitamin C, and herbal or homeopathic combination formulas are extremely helpful when it comes to killing yeast. Alternative therapies such as colon hydrotherapy and FIR Infrared heat therapy will help to remove yeast die-off quicker than your body will do it on its own. I have found that when colloidal silver is used in treating yeast, people do not seem to get the "die-off" symptoms that commonly feel flu-like.

One of the most important things you can do to prevent systemic yeast overgrowth is to supplement with probiotics (healthy bacteria) on a regular basis, but especially when finishing a course of antibiotics. So if you suffer from bloating, sugar cravings, sensitivity to smells, bad breath or body odor, athlete's foot, jock itch, thick cloudy toe nails, joint pain or hard to diagnose skin rashes, be very suspicious of a yeast invasion. It is most likely there.

A very typical scenario is detailed in Chapter 2. Lizzy is one of hundreds I see with the same classic symptoms of yeast over-growth.

Back to the Colon…

Peristalsis is the contraction of the smooth muscle that is essential to propel digestive wastes through the intestinal tract. An analogy would be how an earthworm propels in order to move through its environment. Peristalsis is essential to having proper bowel movements, preventing a back "log" of toxic waste. Habitual laxative users beware—the longer you have been on laxatives the less your body is able to perform normal peristalsis. Your colon function may essentially burn out. Well-chewed fruits, vegetables, seeds and nuts are a great way to facilitate peristalsis in the colon. What about fiber products, you say? Be very careful, because as you will read in the upcoming chapters, fiber supplements will most likely backfire on you if you already suffer from constipation.

One of my favorite healing gurus is Bernard Jensen (1908-2001). Dr. Jensen had seen more than 350,000 patients over the course of his 60-year healing career as a chiropractor, iridologist, colon therapist and author. He established healing facilities that were responsible for turning the health of his patients around when all seemed hopeless. His books, now ancient gems of wisdom, have been some of the most educational and helpful books that I have read. Dr. Jensen, in my opinion, had some of the best philosophies and visions when it came to the body, nutrition and healing. One of his main organs of focus when it came to true health and healing was the colon. Dr. Jensen viewed the colon as a sewage system. When it is clean and functioning properly, we are happy and well. When our diets are lacking of real food and nutrition, this sewer becomes more like a cesspool that remains within us. Over time, things stagnate, ferment and putrefy. This will most likely lead to Leaky Gut Syndrome, also referred to as autointoxication.

Autointoxication is defined as a state of being poisoned by toxic substances produced within the body. When the digestive system doesn't work properly, autointoxication results. This happens when food begins to break down without being eliminated. Proteins putrefy and rot, carbohydrates ferment, and oils and fats turn rancid. The body becomes poisoned from its own waste. Many constipated individuals fail to see this side of the story, as constipation is viewed solely as an uncomfortable inconvenience.

One of Dr. Jensen's teachers was Dr. Harvey Kellogg, who spent much of his life studying the colon. Dr. Kellogg believed that 90 percent of all disease is due to an improperly functioning colon. Years ago the National College in Chicago performed over 300 autopsies. Patient history revealed that 285 of them had regular bowel habits, and the small remainder of that study claimed to be constipated. Ironically, autopsies revealed that the majority of those autopsied had been chronically constipated. Some had a colon diameter of 12 inches; remember that a normal diameter is approximately 2.5 inches.

I would love to see medical schools go a little bit deeper in their dissection of the cadaver in their anatomy training. I find it very funny that when I mention parasites to physicians, they look at me as if I am crazy. So I asked one of the medical students, "When you dissect the colon, what do you see? Do you measure it? Weigh it? Examine the contents?" Surprisingly, the student informed me that the colon was not dissected at all. Wow, we are missing a whole bunch of information here!

I would personally want to know the weight, shape and diameter of each section. How much fecal matter was found—how much did it weigh? Parasites? Why isn't anyone looking at this when the health of the colon dictates our health? This is possibly my next project for another day.

Leaky Gut Syndrome is a term you are not likely to hear from your primary care provider or gastroenterologist, but there is plenty of evidence to make this a very real issue that needs attention. Leaky Gut Syndrome, or to be medically appropriate, intestinal permeability, is a result of damage to the lining of the intestinal wall. Chronic constipation combined with a diet lacking in nutrients will predispose any individual to this unfortunate condition. It compromises the health of all internal organs. Harmful bacteria, incompletely digested proteins and fats, along with other toxic debris, are all able to penetrate the fragile and damaged lining causing a host of unwanted symptoms. This may trigger an autoimmune reaction that can be as mild as some intestinal bloating and gas, to much more severe conditions such as fatigue, joint pain, skin conditions and other inflammatory conditions. An abnormal number of allergies are very common with this condition. If you are becoming intolerant to more and more foods, you may very well be suffering from Leaky Gut Syndrome.

Leaky Gut Syndrome is what I believe Dr. Jensen refers to when he describes symptoms of a poorly functioning colon. Mental depression, listlessness, bad breath, and pale skin with dark circles under the eyes are toxic red flags that something is not right. If left to their own course, these symptoms turn into premature aging and a brain that cannot see through the sluggishness to enjoy life. For me, and hopefully you as well, your life is about quality, as we have no guarantees on the quantity.

Irritable Bowel Syndrome (IBS) is an overly used blanket diagnosis that is given to anyone who has digestive woes. From diarrhea to constipation, gas and bloating, IBS is a very loose term for "yeah, yeah you have some sort of bowel issue and we're not sure how to fix you."

What is a healthy bowel movement supposed to look like anyway? I get this question all the time. This is how I would describe a healthy movement: Light brown in color. Color is largely determined by diet. The more animal protein in the diet, the darker it may be. Soft. A healthy bowel movement leaves the body in less time than it takes to empty your bladder—without straining! (Got most of you here—didn't I?) Breaks apart easy. Not that I want you all to stir the pot, so to say. But if you did, your fecal waste should fall apart easily. No plungers needed.

If your poop resembles bunny pellets, ribbons or a rock, this book was written for you. If you alternate between constipation and liquid explosions, this book is for you as well. Mucous that resembles seaweed or white slime is typical in those with food allergies and/or parasites. Straining to have a bowel movement is not normal and will most likely lead to hemorrhoids down the road if you don't already have them.

Constipation Defined

By medical definition, constipation is an acute or chronic condition in which bowel movements occur less often than usual or consist of hard, dry stools that are painful or difficult to pass. Bowel habits vary, but an adult who has not had a bowel movement in three days or a child who has not had a bowel movement in four days is considered constipated.

I hope you are not ready to close this book as you

fail to meet the criteria of being "constipated" by medical definition. Reading further will potentially add quality years to your life and prove that the above criteria are far too generous. Two to four days without a bowel movement is unacceptable and unfortunate. Bowel movements should occur at least twice daily if you are eating healthy. Once is typically not enough. Some of my most severely constipated clients are the ones who insist they move daily.

How can you eat three to four times daily and move your bowels just once a day, or heaven forbid, every few days? Constipation is common in all age groups, and as you will learn from this book, there are many contributing factors that may predispose some individuals. If left ignored, constipation usually escalates and can also lead the individual to a host of other ailments.

Hemorrhoids

Hemorrhoids are defined as a mass of dilated veins and swollen tissue around the anus. They can be internal, external or both. Most often the underlying cause is chronic constipation—years of it. Pelvic congestion is typically the cause of hemorrhoids. Pregnancy is a non-pathologic element that may predispose women to hemorrhoids, even if they are not constipated. Sadly, many individuals opt for surgical hemorrhoid removal (hemorrhoidectomy) rather than clear up the cause of the problem—constipation. Because this is a very painful procedure to recover from, pain medications are needed. The irony of this is that pain medications are notorious for constipating people. If the constipation issue is not addressed, collateral circulation is reestablished and the vicious cycle is sure to begin again. Medicine today is inadequate when it comes to helping those with chronic constipation.

Mirilax (polyethylene glycol 3350) and "eat more fiber" is typically the best you're going to get as far as help goes. The Mirilax may help initially, but over time you will need more and more. This is just another common Band-Aid remedy in medicine, without addressing the reason or cause of the constipation in the first place.

I highly recommend that you do not take fiber supplements if you are constipated, unless you enjoy that bloated, "I'm going to blow up" feeling. Stick to raw fruits, vegetables, nuts and seeds. These are the best forms of fiber. Besides the discomfort, chronic constipation predisposes us to a large number of diseases and degenerative conditions, including cancer.

I Know I Am Constipated!

So you know you are constipated—congratulations! You will have an easier time finding what works than the majority of the population that still does not know that they are walking around constipated. As you get through this book you will slowly gather information and remedies that will assist you in making chronic constipation a thing of the past. What you may not have considered is that many individuals that suffer, suffer constipation due to emotional reasons as well as physical ones. This will also be considered and addressed as we move through your learning process.

Sadly, many areas of your life are affected, as constipation leaves you worrying about travel, how your clothes will fit, and God forbid you pass gas at the most inopportune time—as many constipated individuals do. You worry about when the urge will strike, because heaven help you if you miss that golden window of "poopertunity" that leaves you doomed for another day.

Passing gas is a very healthy and common biological function; but in the constipated individual, it may tend to be loud and accompanied by the most obnoxious smells—as compared to a person with a healthier colon function.

Many of you have learned to resist the urge to move your bowels, as the timing is not appropriate (according to you). This bad habit often begins during childhood when school-age children feel shy about asking to go to the bathroom. Many of my clientele will not have a bowel movement in public places, making chronic constipation very difficult to cure. This is a mental handicap that needs to be dealt with in order to *Free Yourself from a Constipated Life.*

If it is the smell you are worried about, there are many purse-size deodorants or even drops that are excellent in eliminating odor. If your hang-up is about possibly passing gas, more commonly know as farting, I'd like to introduce you to the famous children's book, *The Gas We Pass: The Story of Farts*, written by Shinta Cho. I keep a copy of this book in my office for my colonic clients to read.

Avoiding your body's urge to move your bowels only sets you up for some painful experiences. Have you ever experienced the stabbing pain of a crooked fart (slang for trapped air within your impacted colon)? Many will tell you they were doubled over in such pain that it sent them to the emergency room, sure that they were going to die. A few hours later they sheepishly exited the hospital after hearing that their colon was full of stool and they just need a good bowel movement (for which they didn't get much help with).

A constipated child should never be ignored! Please do what you can to remedy this situation while they are young. At the very least there are chewable probiotics to be taken daily and aloe capsules that can be put into food on occasion. This works well for most children along with the removal of gluten and dairy in some cases.

Unfortunately the traditional medical establishment is not very helpful when it comes to helping individuals with constipation. "Take fiber," they say. Fiber supplements will typically make constipation worse. If you are already constipated, how is a bulking agent going to make things flow? OUCH!

I Poop Daily—I'm Not Constipated!

When I initially meet people for consultations or colon hydrotherapy, many will insist that they are not constipated. "I go every day," they say with conviction. Then I get them on the table and nothing moves. They typically think—"I must just be empty," until they hit the bathroom and eliminate half of their body weight in old, petrified fecal matter. I am exaggerating, but to the individual, it feels amazing. They are shocked, to say the least, but feel great as they leave the appointment. This usually is what needs to take place before I can convince someone that they are constipated.

Now you don't have to have a colonic in order to have this revelation. If your diet contains breads, processed foods, and you typically eat 3-4 times per day, two bowel movements are minimal requirements. Any less than that, you, my friend, are holding. Because your state of constipation has most likely occurred very gradually over an extended period of time, there is no pain. The condition is not acute and you are not likely to think anything is wrong. So what's the problem, you say? Eventually this accumulates and as you will learn in the next chapter, you may be suffering symptoms and have not even given the possibility of constipation a thought. My advice to you is to keep the possibility open that yes, even you, may be constipated and there is always room for improvement.

Chapter 2

Symptoms of CONSTIPATION

C onstipation has many faces, as you soon shall see. The following symptoms and scenarios may surprise you, but I bet you fit in there somewhere. The personal stories are my favorite. I am forever grateful to those who contributed.

Oh My Aching Belly

I initially begin my colon therapy session with a massage of the abdomen. This usually helps to get things moving for us in order to make the most of our time together. Many times, I wince more than the client, as I cannot believe they are not walking in pain based on what I feel. It is easy to feel a full colon, especially when there is constipation. It is sometimes at this point during the visit that the client realizes there may be a problem.

Many individuals suffer discomfort at the lower left part of the abdomen. This is typically where most have a problem. As I said earlier, as the digested waste travels through the colon, water absorption takes place. By the time it gets to the left side, just before the designated exit, it has become solid and more difficult to move. By avoiding the urge, it (your poop) is likely to make itself comfortable and stretch things out a bit.

Some have discomfort in different areas. This may in part be due to a narrowing (stricture) in certain parts of the colon. Many who complain of pain below the rib cage that runs horizontally across the abdomen should consider food intolerance and the possibility of Candida or yeast.

Those that feel a mild discomfort on the lower right side of the abdomen should give thought to the possibility of intestinal parasites. This is a very common occurrence (even if you have never left the United States) that I see very often.

Chronic Sinus Conditions

Hey, I thought this was a book about constipation, not sinus issues. Well guess what? Those of you suffering from chronic sinus issues can just assume that your colon is congested as well. Conditions involving abundant mucous are not healthy and will negatively affect your immune system and overall health by slowing the filtration systems within our bodies. Breathing is sluggish, digestion is sluggish, lymphatic drainage is sluggish and of course, pooping becomes sluggish. Many individuals will report mucous in their stools.

Here is a typical scenario that I see at least weekly, and men are just as susceptible as women. I'll call her Lizzy:

I came to Journey II Health to meet with Cathi, for I was at my wits end and was about to go crazy if I did not get relief soon. I'm sure, had I gone to the doctor again, they would have prescribed something for depression or anxiety.

It all started about a year ago. I had a sinus attack that just would not go away. My doctor put me on an antibiotic and a steroid dose pack. Things seemed to be improving so I was happy. Diet was never mentioned. A week later, I developed a horrible yeast infection. I tried to use over-the-counter creams but it seemed persistent so I followed up with my gynecologist. She gave me a Diflucan pill and all was better again for a few weeks.

My sinuses started to bother me again, and although I did not feel like I had a full blown yeast infection, something just did not feel right down there. Well to speed the story up, I had tried 4 different antibiotics, 2 more rounds of steroids and countless treatments for yeast. I felt terrible! Even worse was the 40 extra pounds I had gained over the year! Yes, I said 40 pounds! Not only that, I now was suffering from IBS (Irritable Bowel Syndrome). Sometimes I was constipated and sometimes I was very loose. I was always uncomfortable with bloating. I would look in the mirror and not even recognize myself.

I also began to develop unusual rashes around my neck, my arms and my bikini area. Some of my friends told me to try hydrocortisone creams but that only seemed to make the condition worse.

Not quite suicidal (but almost), I sought out the help of someone who would help me in a natural way. I was tired of the medications and they obviously were not helping. I wanted a more natural approach.

As I met with Cathi, she smiled as I told my story. She listened as I cried and expressed my frustration. My body was out of control and I felt like it was hopeless.

When I was done venting, Cathi looked me straight in the eye and said I can help you and you will be feeling noticeably better in just a few weeks—but it will take time to clear it for good. She made it sound so easy. I was skeptical. Why couldn't my doctor help me?

She proceeded to type my blood, I am an O, and gave me guidelines to follow. No sugar, no wheat, no dairy! Follow the blood type guidelines. She placed me on probiotics (healthy bacteria) as she explained that the multiple antibiotics and steroids had destroyed most of my good bacteria leaving me open to a body full of yeast. She also placed me on colloidal silver and vitamin C and a few other supplements. She seemed so sure of herself. I left the office feeling like there was hope...finally!

Within six weeks, I was down 15 pounds. I could breathe, I wasn't having any IBS symptoms, my skin rashes were completely gone and I felt more energetic than I had in a long time. I am forever grateful.

Sadly, this story is a frequent scenario at my office. In Lizzy's case, the original problem was that she was ingesting too much dairy and wheat products, thinking that was the healthy thing to do. For her blood type, it was the underlying reason for the sinusitis and chronic congestion. The medications wiped out any good bacteria she may have had left and the steroids only made the conditions more favorable for the yeast (Candida) to flourish.

Doctors don't know this, and even those who are open-minded rarely consider diet as the origin of most health issues. They DO want to help you, but unfortunately the only tools in their bags are a variety of medications to help suppress some of your uncomfortable symptoms. These rarely treat the underlying cause.

My Back Is Killing Me

Often times during the course of relieving someone of their constipation, the individual comments on the disappearance of chronic lower back pain. They may have spent years searching therapies, visiting chiropractors and other venues in order to relieve their discomfort.

What I did not learn—or rather—pay much attention to in colon therapy school, was the large number of people who walk around with lower back pain that would be greatly relieved if they experienced a colonic.

I am amazed at the number of people who suffer from chronic lower back pain. Bulging discs, usually L4 & L5, is a common finding on the MRI. Your doctor will suggest physical therapy and maybe even prescribe pain pills. As mentioned earlier, pain pills cause constipation.

Very little focus is placed on the 20 to 40 pounds of excess weight that usually accompanies this condition. Not only would changing the diet facilitate better bowel movements, but the weight loss that would follow is most likely to help resolve the back pain as well.

I'd like to share my findings with you. CLEAN THAT CONSTIPATED COLON AND SAY GOODBYE TO BACK PAIN. These results have repeated themselves over and over and I cannot ignore what I have seen with my own eyes. It makes sense to me that the over-distended colon increases the pressure within the pelvis, affecting nerves and the integrity of the lower lumbar spine. My clients don't come to me to have their back pain taken care of, but often enough, that's exactly what happens. They also don't think that they are constipated as they "go" once a day—but are amazed when they realize what it is like to be truly regular.

I'm not in any way saying colon therapy cures all back pain, but if you are one of the many sufferers, you should consider the possibility of an over-distended constipated colon. Pain medications only add to constipation, making this situation worse and making you want even more medication.

The Constipated Traveler

This is a scenario that I see over and over again, and because I tend to travel frequently, I see what it can do to the individual. They become obsessed with going to the bathroom. If they are attending a conference, they usually cannot sit for long periods of time as they become too uncomfortable. Their attention span becomes less that adequate and many key points of a good conference could be missed.

They will run to the nearest drug or food store searching out the items that will most likely "move" them. Prunes, teas and laxatives may provide them with a few very uncomfortable hours, but eventually the blow out occurs and they are back to their happy, productive and comfortable selves.

God help the poor traveler who is planning on wearing a bathing suit. They just don't feel like putting one on, for fear of looking pregnant. Intimate relations are affected as well. It is very hard to get in the mood or find positions that are comfortable for sex if your belly or back is aching from constipation.

I have actually had patients tell me that they won't travel because this always happens and they feel like a burden to their traveling companions. How sad, especially because with a little planning this could have been avoided. Cape Aloe will always be in my suitcase from this day forward for these types of situations. I will discuss much more on this supplement later.

Parasites? Yikes!

This section is not for the squeamish but contains very valuable information that pertains to at least 85 percent of you. I hope you share with your health care provider if you feel it may be an issue.

If the colon is not evacuated twice a day or more, parasites can breed and cause further symptoms. Common symptoms of parasite infestation include the following: pain in joints and muscles; inability to gain weight; itchy ears, nose and anus; eating more than normal; sugar cravings; nutrient deficiencies and anemia; teeth grinding; and weakened immune function.

I stumbled upon Ann Louise Gittleman at a natural health conference. I realize now how important that stumble-upon was. When Ann Louise began to speak about the prevalence of parasites and the ailments they contribute to, I knew I was learning something valuable. Although she has written many books to date, *Guess What Came to Dinner?* is one of her best works on a topic we should all become a bit more familiar with.

In practice, I have seen worms as tiny as the eye can detect and some over a foot long. I have identified flukes, roundworms and more. To date I have yet to meet the tapeworm up close and personal, but I am sure I have been in the company of many who harbor them.

A few years back I wrote a letter to every gastrointestinal specialist I could find in my local phone book. The funny thing about chronically constipated people is that when you treat them for parasites many of their complaints are alleviated. I felt so sure I was on to something and felt it was my responsibility to share the information.

Five years later, I am absolutely convinced that undiagnosed abdominal pain, many types of Irritable Bowel Syndrome (IBS) and Colitis could easily be eliminated if practitioners would consider parasite treatment. Why don't they? I'm really not sure.

Most of us with dogs treat our furry loved ones at least yearly, if not monthly, for parasites. They eat the same thing daily and we aggressively treat them for worms—what about us? We eat a large variety of foods in comparison to our animals. When was the last time your doctor offered you prophylactic treatment for parasites?

First let me state that most of us have been exposed to parasites at some point in our life. Research has shown that an estimated 85 percent of all American adults are infected with some sort of parasite. More than 100 types of parasitic worms can be living happily in human bodies. Only about five percent of these varieties can be tested positively with only 20 percent accuracy. This means that parasite testing has extremely high false negative results. Constipation is the perfect breeding ground for parasites, yet many medical professionals only consider parasites in cases of diarrhea.

I once had a physician for a professional sports team ask why I would treat his patient for parasites without testing. When I explained that we actually saw them, he had little to say. I know many individuals who have tested negative for parasites, but possess many symptoms that make them likely hosts.

Some parasites are big enough in size that they can be seen by the naked eye, while the others are microscopic in size. Parasites can range from tiny amoebas, which are visible only under a microscope, to tapeworms 3-30 feet in length. Fortunately, the easy-to-eliminate roundworm species are the most common and tapeworm not so common.

Again, many of us can live without parasite drama if we remain constipation free (moving bowels at least twice daily). Once constipated, we give those pesky critters a beautiful environment to flourish. The more toxic we are, the more they love us. Common complaints include lower right abdominal pain, teeth grinding at night (bruxism), and dark circles under the eyes. Grinding of teeth is often misdiagnosed as TMJ (temporomandibular joint disorders), as parasites are more active at night, causing us a restless attempt at sleep.

Many years ago I worked a busy medical/ surgical floor as a staff nurse. We did stool samples for ova (eggs) and parasites all the time. The results were often negative—false negative I would now conclude. As a colon therapist who sees parasites with her own eyes, what I do know is that they are usually not within the fecal sample. They are seen and excreted with a mucous-like coating. Anyone who has bowel movements with mucous strands should be very suspicious.

We are exposed to parasites by eating produce, walking barefoot in the grass, petting a pig, eating fish, and many other circumstances. It is not that we are dirty or contaminated—it is life. Actually it would be very hard to avoid exposure, especially if you eat healthy. But for those who occupy a poor diet and find themselves constipated, you will grow and multiply your parasites faster. Something you may want to consider: cooking does not always kill parasites, but freezing does. As a naturopath, I avoid medications as much as possible. As a midwife, I have the ability to prescribe medication. If one were to eliminate parasites using herbs such as wormwood, black walnut and pumpkin seed, the minimum treatment would be two to six weeks. Although extremely effective, many of my clients are not compliant with the dosing, making their therapy ineffective. Prescribing mebendazole or albendazole for parasites along with colon cleansing has helped hundreds of people who have found no relief in laxatives or doctor visits. Unexplained congestion and skin ailments, just to name a few complaints, can even be cleared.

Carol came to see me after struggling from a lifetime of constipation and stomach issues. Carol is a beautiful schoolteacher in her mid-twenties who looked and carried herself off as healthy. She had seen many specialists who provided little help and felt she was doomed to living in constant discomfort. Here is her story:

I have had tummy troubles for as long as I can remember. I recall being at a Girl Scout meeting and excusing myself to the bathroom because I had sharp pains and lying flat on the floor was the only way I could experience relief. Occurrences like that didn't seem odd, they were just part of my life since childhood.

I have always dealt with constipation. Regardless of diet or lifestyle changes, "poop" never came easy for me. I was always in awe of people who "just went" everyday, like clockwork without intervention. I've tried every laxative, fiber supplement and infomercial special on the market to no avail. Throughout college, I was hospitalized twice for excruciating stomach pain. I never did get any clear answers to what the cause was.

I did see a specialist and was diagnosed with IBS and I was given prescription meds. I took the meds for a short time. I felt like they were a short-term fix of the symptoms, but I didn't understand what the problem was, let alone what should be done to fix it. Again, I just lived with constipation and assumed it was just "how I was".

In 2007, on my wedding day, I suffered massive pulmonary emboli. A blood clot traveled through my heart and burst into three in my lungs. I was lucky to survive and following this life-changing event, I wanted to get myself healthy. My main goal after my marriage was to have children. One change I made to achieve this goal was to tackle the issue of constipation.

I saw Journey II Health opened and I was intrigued. I also noticed a sign for colonics

*in the window. I had a few colonics years
ago but I was not consistent with them. I
went to see Cathi with hopes that she could
help with my chronic constipation. Initially I
was skeptical of the results but I was open
minded and hopeful. Cathi was a great
source of knowledge. She was patient,
comforting and such a positive spirit. She
stuck with me and truly made a difference
for me. I purchased a package of colonics
and decided to stay consistent with
treatment because as "icky" as the process
may have seemed at the time, I was making
progress.*

*Slowly I started to become more regular.
This was an entirely new experience for me.
I attribute the change to the series of
colonics, taking Cape Aloe, getting rid of my
horrifying parasites (gross!) and Cathi's
support. I felt better and healthier than I
had in a long time. The following year I
became pregnant with my son. How ironic
that Cathi happened to be the midwife on
staff when I gave birth to my first child.*

*I have recently given birth to my daughter. I
had amazing, uneventful, easy pregnancies
and deliveries and I truly believe that is a
direct result of a clean colon! I no longer
need regular colonics but I do take Cape
Aloe as needed to stay regular, and it works*

like a charm. I never have to resort to any harsh laxatives.

I don't know if I will ever be one of those regular people who "just go" every morning at the same time, but I sure have come a long way. I feel good, and I monitor myself closely for changes and I know what I need to do to remedy the situation. Colonics were the catalyst for a healthier, happier me!

Carol was one of the more extreme cases I have come across over the years. She came in weekly for at least two to three months. I remember feeling bad about this, as most respond to the therapy in four to six sessions. Carol didn't seem to mind as she sadly stated, "At least I get to go—I always feel better." We both had the opportunity to see at least two twelve-inch parasites during our sessions. A big part of her treatment was ridding her body of the parasites, which I believe with every fiber of my being had something to do with her blood clots. Once the parasite issue was treated, that seemed to be the tipping point for relief.

A diet that frequents bread, sugar and processed foods only helps to maintain an environment that a parasite will flourish in. Unfortunately, the majority of the population eats to support their parasites.

Prevention is the best way to avoid the parasite invasion. A healthy diet with a healthy elimination of minimally two bowel movements daily will not only improve your immune system and overall health, but also make you an undesirable host for parasites. Supplying your colon with a high quality probiotic formula will help to ensure a healthy environment that parasites dislike. Washing your hands before you eat and always after using the bathroom is the most important thing you can do to prevent parasite contamination. Washing your produce very well is a must. Using a half-teaspoon of bleach to a gallon of water and soaking your produce for 15-30 minutes is a very effective way to ensure that you have eliminated parasite contamination without contaminating your food.

Unrefined natural sea salt, fresh lemon and raw garlic have antiseptic properties within the body. Fresh raw pineapple and papaya have strong digestive enzymes that have been used by natives in Mexico to remedy worm infestations.

Parasites hate pumpkins seed, wormwood, black walnut and cloves. There are many effective herbal and homeopathic remedies on the market. If you follow directions, you can be successful in eliminating parasites without the use of prescription drugs.

"Miraculous" is a word that is commonly used when patients report an 85-90 percent improvement in their symptoms. I am all for preventative and proactive treatment against parasites. It just makes sense.

To date, I have not gotten one reply or comment from any of those gastrointestinal specialists. Nevertheless I will continue to practice what has helped hundreds, as my satisfaction comes from their happiness and well-being.

Diarrhea (Doesn't make sense, does it?)

Often, I will see clients who complain of diarrhea more than being constipated. This individual is very easily remedied with the help of probiotics and Calcium Bentonite clay. We clean up their diet, add fiber, and usually send them on their way—easy.

But what I have seen that may surprise you is the very constipated individual who will only have loose stools. This may often come at the most inappropriate of times and many of these people will have embarrassing accidents.

A basic, but easy to understand explanation goes like this: When the liquid products of digestion pass through the ileocecal valve that connects the small intestine to the large intestine, it is looking to be absorbed and solidified as it travels the length of the large intestine. When the majority of that space is taken up by old stool and putrefying mucous, it has nowhere to go but out. This usually comes with little warning. So the complaint is that they have diarrhea, not constipation. Once the colon is cleaned out, diet is modified, and healthy bacteria colonies are established, things will usually return to normal.

Bad Breath & Other Body Odors

We've all suffered from bad breath at one time or another, but some individuals suffer on a continual basis. Those suffering chronically should consider the possibility of internal toxicity. These individuals are likely to suffer from body and foot odor as well.

Bad breath, otherwise know as halitosis, is estimated to affect up to 50 percent of the population in varying degrees. Bad breath can be caused by a variety of conditions. Poor oral hygiene, oral abscesses, and gingivitis can harbor odor-inducing bacteria that may cause bad breath. Flossing daily, brushing at least twice daily, and eating raw fruits and vegetables can improve this situation.

Unfortunately, most people suffering from bad breath have issues that lie far deeper than the oral cavity. A study in the Journal of Medical Microbiology suggests that H. pylori can be an underlying cause of bad breath, as well as the more common association to stomach ulcers. Another frequent correlation is chronic constipation.

Chronically constipated people typically suffer from Candida and/or an abundance of unhealthy bacteria in relation to friendly, health promoting bacteria. This is often the bad breath that no gum or mouthwash can conquer. Morning breath is a given and unfortunately, most will ignore the gentle hints given by loved ones or co-workers.

Other causes may be related to upper respiratory infections. Bronchitis, sinusitis, and even colds break down tissue, starting a flow of cells and mucous that feed the bacteria, which create foul odors. Medications such as antidepressants and diuretics can dry the mouth, predisposing the individual to bad breath.

Those who have tried the carbohydrate restricting Atkins diet know all too well the bad breath that is associated with a high protein intake and ketoacidosis. People who ingest large quantities of dairy or sugar are more prone to "yeasty" type odors. Those who skip breakfast set themselves up for bad-breath potential. Uncontrolled diabetes, anemia, kidney disease, liver disease, and excessive alcohol consumption are also contributing factors.

If you or a loved one suffers from chronic bad breath, there are some remedies that may be helpful.

- Clean the colon.

- Brush with baking soda or a hydrogen peroxide containing toothpaste. Toothpaste with xylitol actually prevents that "bad" bacterium from sticking to your teeth and gums. Chewing gum with xylitol is not a bad idea. These three ingredients make it difficult for bacteria to grow.

- Alleviate constipation through diet and supplementation. Cape Aloe is a very safe, gentle and effective stool-softening agent. We will go into much more detail later.

- Probiotic (healthy bacteria) supplements will help create an environment that minimizes foul smelling bacteria and yeast.

- Supplements containing chlorophyll help to deodorize the body from the inside out. Adding large amounts chlorophyll rich vegetable juices to our diets is like getting a blood and organ cleanser by washing our bodies from the inside out. Chlorophyll is known as an internal healer. In fact there are many, many benefits. Chlorophyll comes in liquid or capsules that are easy to take.

- Minimize refined carbohydrate and sugar consumption. Bad, odor-causing bacteria flourish in this environment.

- Parsley, mint leaves, lemon and avocado all have breath-improving benefits. Individuals who eat greens such as spinach, kale, beet greens and wheatgrass, or include green supplements in their daily diet, are unlikely to suffer from halitosis.

- All-natural mouthwashes (no fluoride) that contain essential oils such as peppermint, thyme, eucalyptus and wintergreen are far more effective than commercial mouthwashes.

- Neem oil has worked on a few people I have worked with. Neem is a vegetable oil that can be found in gel caps. It works as a deodorizing agent in the gastrointestinal tract.

I'll stick to my guns and say you are what you eat, digest, and hold on to. People who have two bowel movements per day rarely suffer from bad breath. By keeping your digestive system healthy and eating a diet that includes plenty of vegetables, you will make bad breath a thing of the past. If not for yourself, consider doing it for those around you.

The Foggy Thinker

Brain fog is a term used to describe feelings of mental dullness or lack of mental clarity. If you feel as if your thoughts are clouded, you may be suffering, and it may be due to your state of internal health, or rather, lack of.

Most individuals who suffer from brain fog are forgetful and because of this, often become discouraged and depressed. Food, hydration and elimination are most likely the biggest contributors but many medications or a hormone imbalance can contribute to foggy thinking as well. Although a sluggish bowel is the likely suspect, B-12 deficiency should be ruled out.

Brain fog is not viewed as a clinical diagnosis, because it cannot be clearly defined by symptoms and cannot be cured with a medication. The individual typically knows they are not functioning well but it is often taken lightly. Brain fog affects adults as well as children. It affects school and work performance. This could then have a trickle-down effect onto interpersonal relationships. All areas of one's life can be negatively affected.

There are many theories that attempt to explain the causes of brain fog. Many believe that heavy metal toxicity is a likely suspect—especially excess copper. Thyroid imbalances have also been blamed. Many who suffer symptoms of hypothyroidism are also constipated. In practice, I have seen symptoms of brain fog completely eliminated through diet and the reestablishment of healthy bowel habits.

Bowel toxicity results from improperly digested food that putrefies, rots and ferments within the large intestine. Over time this will slowly poison our liver as well as other organs. Many individuals today have elevated liver enzymes or have been diagnosed with "fatty liver disease". This is most likely a result of a colon gone wrong. Most of these individuals will also report foggy thinking.

Diet is an aggravating factor that will be addressed

in more detail in the upcoming chapters. Gluten, sugar and food additives are contributing factors for brain fog and other issues related to constipation.

Worst Case Scenario

When you see the commercials on TV for any type of drug, you'll notice that they quickly ramble through a list of side effects that you would think no one in their right mind would want to experience. Even with death being one of the side effects, the desperate person who does not feel well will most likely give it a try.

I have seen constipation almost take the life of someone I care about very deeply. Now I'm not trying to scare you, but there are some of you out there who truly scare me. Unfortunate stories of a week or more between bowel movements are on the extreme side of what I see. This individual scares me as I can only imagine the internal toxicity. To my lack of understanding, these individuals present life-long stories of constipation and trips to the emergency department or gastroenterologist, only to find little help in the long term.

Most often these individuals look fairly healthy— they are typically not overweight, have tried cleaning up their diet, and have tried all supplements associated with constipation. They may be typically blown-off by the medical establishment as they do not appear to be clinically sick. This is a set up, in my experience, for what I consider the worst-case scenario.

Anne is a woman I had met at a local health fair. She is an incredible artist and photographer. We became friends and I began my attempt to help her with what I would consider horrific constipation. Anne could go two weeks between bowel movements and had very little appetite because of this. She experienced abdominal discomfort almost constantly.

We began a series of colon hydrotherapy sessions in the hopes of reestablishing regular bowel habits. I was not sure how effective we would be at bringing back peristalsis and normal colon function, but at the very least, she would leave my office feeling so much better than when she walked in.

Typically when initiating a series of colon hydrotherapy sessions, we schedule at least three to six sessions that are no further than a week apart. Anne lived at least an hour from my office, making it difficult to come for regular visits.

Anne received about five to six colonics before she began to respond well. After two months of treatments, Anne was having regular bowel movements on her own. She reported feeling much better.

Because Anne also lived in another part of the country for half the year, I went almost a year before I saw her again. She came in to photograph some items for me as we were working on a catalog together. She mentioned to me that she had not gone to the bathroom in weeks and even had no movement after drinking a half bottle of castor oil. Castor oil internally would cause a dramatic blow out of the colon—something I do not recommend. I was stunned when she told me this and was more than a little concerned. "We need to fix this soon," I thought to myself.

Two days later I received a phone call from one of Anne's dearest friends. She informed me that Anne had been rushed to the hospital in the middle of the night with severe stomach pain and was rushed to surgery. The surgeon removed a large portion of her colon as it was constipated and gangrene. Gangrene is a term that describes a serious and potentially life threatening condition that arises when a mass of body tissue dies (necrosis). Anne's condition was severe; a large portion of her colon was dead! I went to visit her a few days later. She did not look well, and was having difficulty breathing. I called out to the nurses' station to have someone check her, and all I know is that a few physician phone calls were made.

Sometime during the night, Anne had a bleeding event that had her sent right back into the operating room. This time she did not wake up. She was kept in the intensive care unit in a drug-induced coma for the next two months. There were so many nights I would return from visiting the ICU that I just thought there was not much hope.

Anne seemed to suffer every possible complication and yet she did wake up to spring in Western New York. I would tease her that it was a heck of a way to avoid winter in Buffalo. The human body never ceases to amaze me.

Six months later she had her colostomy reversed and is now trying to enjoy a normal life. Recovery from extended periods of a comatose state can be very difficult. Things we take for granted need to be learned all over again. Breathing, eating, walking and even thinking all have to be relearned. Sometimes this can take years.

Death would actually be the worst case scenario, but seeing those who love Anne suffer in the uncertainty of her condition and outcome for two months was close enough. A story of constipation gone wrong—Anne's story:

I have suffered with poor digestive health all of my life. It wasn't until my early 20's that I sought to find help from a specialist. It wasn't easy but I subjected myself to a rectal exam by a very handsome young doctor who sent me off to my first colonoscopy. I followed through only to find out that my colon looked great except for a couple of small polyps. His advice was to treat me for IBS, (Metamucil at that time) and come back in 3 years. After the second colonoscopy and complaints about pain in my abdomen, he ordered a CT scan. Even the scans came up with nothing conclusive. "Come back in 3 years, and again, take something similar to Metamucil." This continued for 20 years.

I continued to ask questions, do research, see my doctor and still there was no real reason behind my sluggish and painful digestive tract. I learned to live with very little relief and made myself the brunt of the family jokes. No one really knew what to do. My mother was a nurse so she helped with advice for using fleet enemas, prune juice, and proper diet. We were all amazed that nothing ever really helped. The poor digestion led to swollen glands and migraine headaches. I eventually ended up with poor adrenal health that led to hyperactive thyroid disease.

The only true relief that I ever found was homeopathic remedies, which I spent a great deal of time researching. I started work with a colon therapist who gave me tremendous relief. In fact I was amazed at how quickly and effectively we managed to cleanse my very sluggish colon.

My mom was a bit angry at the prospect but I assured her that it was fine as long as we were getting results. When I found out that this particular office was not professionally trained, I backed off. I did finally find Cathi at Journey II Health and after some time, found relief again. I just could not remain consistent as I traveled.

By the time I got into my late 40's, all bets were off. Nothing was working properly and it was beginning to show. I tried cleanses that friends recommended however some of them had the reverse effects and didn't touch my problem.

This progressed with no help from my primary care doctors or my specialists. One day I was rushed to the hospital with intense pain that ended up being a twisted bowel. Actually a very sick, twisted bowel. The surgeon took out the infected area and re-sectioned me. Unfortunately he should have given me an ileostomy because the re-section came apart. I was leaking for 8 days until they took me back into surgery. Two months later after a long and difficult stay in ICU, I was lucky enough to go home.

My case is rare but it is worth noting. What you need to realize is that it is not okay to go through life constipated. The long-term effects of poor colon health are dangerous and often fatal. Please pay attention to the signs in your life and in the lives of your children that may begin at a very early age.

Anne and I have met a few times again since her recovery to discuss the physical and emotional healing that has been taking place. Her perspective of the time she was in a coma is described as a beautiful symphony of prayers, those of which she heard in many languages at the same time. She emphasized that the person in a coma does hear. She also describes seeing—or rather—feeling me from the upper corner of the room, not the bed. Anne wants me to relay to the reader, and to all that care for those in a comatose state, that your presence and energy is felt. She describes these things with such beauty.

It is my hope that this experience comforts others who may be facing similar situations.

Chapter 3

You Are What You Eat

There is no way to get around it! No pill, no supplement, no exercise—nothing. You cannot out-supplement poor eating habits. Period. The sad reality is that most individuals do not know what healthy eating is. They continue to reach for the artificial sweeteners, the labels of "low-fat" and "sugar-free", not realizing that they are accelerating aging and degeneration within their body. Low-fat products are typically high in sugar, while low-sugar and sugar-free items are loaded with chemicals that no body should be exposed to.

Children are being raised on colored sugar water and macaroni and cheese from a box. Prepackaged lunch meals contain no benefit, but do give our children a healthy dose of what constipates them—wheat and dairy. We are seeing incredible numbers of children with behavior and learning disabilities. If you don't think that what your child eats has anything to do with behavioral issues, you are sadly misinformed. I am in awe of what people put in their shopping carts; if they only knew.

Many books have been written on the topics

discussed below. I'm just giving you a glance.

SUGAR Dilemma

The Average American consumes over 170 pounds of sugar a year. 18.2 million people in the United States have been diagnosed with diabetes. It is estimated that 5.2 million people are unaware that they have it.

Parents are virtually pouring sugar down their children's throats in the form of juice boxes, fast foods and sugary snacks. No parent would intentionally hurt their own child, but that is exactly what is happening when you allow your children to consume and become addicted to these foods. Diets high in sugar are typically low in omega-3 fatty acids, which are common denominators in children diagnosed with ADHD (Attention Deficit Hyperactive Disorder). Childhood obesity is an epidemic and has more to do with what we are feeding our children than a lack of exercise.

Most are shocked when I reveal to them that they are consuming sugar every time they put something in their mouth. Sports drinks, canned soups, bottled salad dressings, peanut butter, protein bars, yogurt, alcohol, bagels and fast foods are just a few examples. Consuming sugar causes your body to hold fat, not lose it.

Foods that contain excess sugar contribute to constipation and obesity. A trap I see many individuals fall into is buying products that state "low fat". Check the sugar content. Typically, low fat items contain more sugar. Fat doesn't make you fat, sugar does!

Imagine Life Without BREAD

For so many individuals, bread is not only a daily habit, but it shows up at almost every meal. Sandwiches, wraps, crackers, bagels, cereal, pizza and pasta are an unfortunate addition to the daily diet and are a significant contribution to the obesity epidemic today.

With a high percentage of the population suffering from gluten sensitivities, we would all benefit from minimizing, or even better, eliminating, bread products from our diet. If you suffer from bloating and allergies, I would venture to bet that if you eliminated all bread products for two weeks, you would feel dramatically better in a variety of ways.

First off, you may notice that your chronic sinus condition that is blamed on the trees, pollen and hay fever will begin to fade away and you may even forget to take your medications. Those suffering from fibromyalgia and brain fog could also see improvement. Next, that extra two inches on the waist will melt off and you won't likely feel bloated after meals and need to undo that top button. These are just external changes you will notice.

Internally, your digestive tract that was likely to be gummed up on a regular basis is now free flowing. Foods will be broken down with greater ease, and the nutrients from the healthy, well chewed foods are able to be absorbed with improved delivery of essential vitamins and minerals. Natural fiber intake from fruits and vegetables will have a broom-like effect on the colon. This will help many who suffer from chronic constipation, as well as an improvement of overall health.

I've actually had people ask me what do I eat if I don't eat bread. Really? Anyone who knows or works with me knows I usually have fresh produce or a variety of salads that I make. Sometimes I use Romaine lettuce leaves as a wrap for tuna, quinoa or egg salads. For dinner—fish, chicken or beef with a vegetable and salad will fill me up. Preparation is key, as I cannot leave the hospital and don't leave my office to go to lunch. If I can do it, anyone can. Your shopping list is likely to change, and in order to eat fresh you will be shopping more frequently and in smaller amounts.

I feel that the food pyramid fails us when it comes to staying healthy and avoiding obesity. Six to twelve servings of grains are the recommended amount. I'd feel like a cow—no thank you! Michelle Obama recently changed the food pyramid to "MyPlate". The plate is split into four sections for fruit, vegetables, grains and protein. A smaller circle sits beside it for dairy products. While this may be an improvement over the food pyramid, it needs to be more specific. With approximately 80 percent of the nation being gluten sensitive, eliminating wheat would benefit most.

Restricting carbohydrates is not the goal. We absolutely need carbohydrates to function properly and maintain adequate energy levels throughout the day. The healthiest carbohydrates are those found in nature. Fruits, vegetables and beans (legumes) are excellent carbohydrate choices. Healthy, gluten-free, whole grains such as steel-cut oats, quinoa, millet and rice make excellent additions to salads as well as side dishes for main meals. There are so many easy and delicious recipes available at your fingertips via the Internet. For those not online, the library will likely have recipe books for gluten-free living.

The downside of life without bread will likely be

the cost of a new wardrobe due to your waist size that is likely to shrink as a result of sticking with this. For those of you with gluten sensitivities, the longer you eliminate wheat products completely, the more likely that they won't be bothersome on a rare occasion. Minimally six months is needed to make your body less reactive. You may, however, feel so much better that you do not want to add them back into your diet.

If nothing else, please become more conscious of how much bread you are consuming. I am sure you will be surprised. Give your body the benefit of bread-free living and see how good you can feel.

The DAIRY Disaster

Of all the food allergies in the US, dairy affects the largest number of people with the most acute symptoms. From colicky babies (a breastfeeding mom passes on her sensitivities), ear infections and tonsillitis, to bloating and chronic sinusitis, dairy allergies affect the lives of millions. Many people, especially children, are needlessly placed on many rounds of antibiotics for symptoms of dairy allergies.

How many people do you know that are "lactose intolerant"? I bet you know more than a few. I also know that the majority of people who suspect they may have a red-flag warning of a dairy allergy will continue to ignore their body's warning signals. Some will even take or drink lactaid in order to continue consuming something that their body clearly does not want. Chronic sinus conditions, along with bloating, gas, diarrhea and even constipation, become normal and frequent complaints tolerated by the individual with a dairy intolerance.

Because we have been brainwashed to believe that dairy is essential for optimal bone health, we continue to suffer. I hope I am not the first to tell you that drinking milk does very little to prevent osteoporosis or even remotely promote health. Cow dairy is extremely hard for humans to digest. 100 percent of humans are allergic to casein, a milk protein. Casein (the main ingredient in Elmer's glue) causes a histamine reaction in most individuals and causes an increase in mucous production. Mucous clogs the works! No one feels good or benefits from excess production.

No other population on the planet consumes more calcium than American women and yet we have, by far, the highest rate of osteoporosis in the world. A study funded by the US National Dairy Council gave a group of postmenopausal women three 8-ounce glasses of skimmed milk per day for two years. They then compared their bones with those women who did not drink milk. The dairy group consumed 1,400mg of calcium per day, and yet lost bone density at twice the rate of the control group (women who did not drink milk).

The Harvard Nurses' Health Study found that women who consumed the most calcium from dairy foods broke more bones than those who rarely drank milk. Milk makes you acidic! Being acidic robs your bones, leaving them brittle and prone to fractures. The majority of Asian populations eat little to no dairy. Most of their calcium comes from vegetable and seaweed sources. Osteoporosis in China is very uncommon.

We are the only mammals that consume dairy once we are weaned from mother's milk. It is just not natural to consume dairy, and it is certainly not healthy. There are, however, better options. Goat milk is easier to digest than cows' milk. Raw milk, although difficult to find, is the superior form of dairy and will not cause allergic reactions in most individuals.

Most individuals consume yogurt on a daily basis. Unfortunately, most consumed yogurts barely qualify as food. Artificial sweeteners and flavorings that are added to many of the popular brands make the majority of the yogurt just another form of junk food. Those eating high quality "real" yogurt with live, active cultures may not find it difficult to digest, as lactose is broken down by healthy, lactic acid bacteria.

Many individuals also suffer from iron deficiency anemia. What few realize is that consuming dairy contributes to iron deficiency, because it blocks iron uptake. Eliminating dairy and increasing greens in the diet usually benefits those with iron deficiency anemia. Wheatgrass, spinach, kale, endive, and beet greens are a few examples of foods that will help raise iron levels faster than any iron pill I know of, without the side effects of constipation and stomach upset. Please note that gluten sensitivities may also be responsible for anemia.

For those of you who want options for your cereal or warm beverage, there are healthy options that actually don't taste bad at all. Rice milk, almond milk and even hemp seed milk are all readily available at your grocery store. These milk alternatives are a great option and a great first step in making healthier choices; just beware of added sugar in some brands. You are probably wondering why I did not mention soy. Many individuals are allergic and it has also become an overly processed food. If you have an "A" blood type, you may be an exception.

Try eliminating ALL dairy products for two

weeks. Not only are you likely to breath easier, feel great, and move your bowels better—you are also likely to drop a few pounds.

FAUX FOOD: Our National Downfall

Most individuals fall for words like "all natural", "heart healthy", and pretty pictures of fruits and vegetables when shopping for groceries. These very misleading marketing ploys are partially responsible for the rising numbers of those diagnosed with heart disease, diabetes, and people suffering from obesity, even though they are eating foods that claim to benefit their health.

A popular fiber bar on the market boasts that a diet high in fiber will help you lose weight and feel full. This oat and chocolate "naturally flavored" bar has more chocolate than oats, and has at least six types of sugar in the ingredient list. If you'd like to experience abdominal bloating and gas from the sugar alcohols, and fast track yourself to an adult onset diabetes diagnosis—eat these!

For children, please do not fall for pictures of fruits or added vitamins on the labels. It infuriates me that many of these products are being sold to the parents of growing children, and we wonder why we see so many suffer from ADD/ADHD and obesity. "Juice" treats that are manufactured by companies famous for making baby food are a perfect example of nutrition gone wrong for toddler age children. There is absolutely NO healthy fat or protein, just 17 grams of sugar and corn syrup.

For those still convinced that eating low-fat will protect their hearts, many fat-free salad dressings have seven or more grams of sugar in the form of high fructose corn syrup. Diabetes first, then heart disease is sure to follow.

Do I really need to mention foods like canned soup, whipped cream products, and cheese foods that resemble plastic more than they do foods? Drinks that are loaded with colors and chemicals, such as sodas and powdered or crystal drinks have no health or protective benefits—they actually hurt you. People come to me all the time in hopes of preventing or curing their illness. If you don't look at the diet first, you are sure to fail in your desire to heal. There is no medication or supplement that will remedy a poor diet!

For those already suffering from diabetes, the old recommendations were to eat sugar-free. How about a slice of sugar-free devil's food cake? You may find yourself running for the bathroom from the laxative effect of maltitol (sugar alcohol), suffering the negative effects from trans fats (partially hydrogenated soybean oil), and let's not forget brain or neurologic damage from sucralose or acesulfame potassium (artificial sweeteners).

Take a good look around you. On average, those that consume diet beverages are at least twenty pounds heavier than those who don't. Artificial sweeteners just create a ravaging sweet tooth in those who consume them. I'll give you my story.

Many years ago, I, weighing all of 130lbs, decided that 16 calories was just too much to be adding to my coffee. God forbid—16 calories! So I proceeded to do the "smart" thing and use a zero-calorie sweetener instead. Because of the extreme sweetness, all I could use was a quarter of a packet. Over the years, I began to add a bit more, for reasons I don't know. By the time I started to read about the dangers, I was ¾ of a packet in. I very slowly added about 10-15lbs to my body over time. It was a hard habit to break—really, it was. Funny thing though, six weeks after I gave up the artificial sweetener I was down almost ten pounds. Nothing else had changed. All the artificial sweeteners had done was make me fatter and probably killed some brain cells.

Katy was a woman who came to see me in hopes of losing some weight and help with her pre-diabetic condition. She insisted she did not have a sweet tooth, but then proceeded to tell me that she loads her coffee with three packets of Splenda (sucralose). YUK! That is the equivalent to approximately 12 teaspoons of sugar. She had a monster sweet tooth and probably suffered migraine headaches as well.

Now, for those who are too busy to cook and must resort to buying frozen meals, know this: Nothing nutritious is cooked in the microwave. Many popular frozen dinners contain more than 50 ingredients and most are downright toxic. A popular brand of frozen chicken with basil cream sauce contains trans fats (partially hydrogenated or hydrogenated anything), chicken parts (you don't want to know), MSG (disguised as whey protein concentrate), and many other chemicals and sugars.

MSG affects many individuals with symptoms such as migraine headaches, upset stomach, fuzzy thinking, diarrhea, heart irregularities, asthma and/or mood swings. MSG (monosodium glutamate) is not easily recognized, as it is hidden under many names. The following ingredients should always be treated as MSG; anything with the word "glutamate", yeast extract, anything "hydrolyzed", autolyzed yeast, gelatin, textured protein, soy protein isolate, soy protein concentrate, whey protein isolate, vetsin, Accent, and ajinomoto. Bouillon and broth often contain MSG and the same goes for soy sauce. Even foods labeled as organic can contain high amounts of sugar and other ingredients that are not health promoting. So many well-intending people are falling for marketing tricks that do not benefit your health. Many are just still stuck in the old thinking that a low-fat sugar-free diet is best, when the exact opposite is true. Look at the cancer rates since the turn of the century; they have escalated tremendously with the addition of food chemicals and preservatives.

Eat foods as they come from nature, in their purest forms. There is such an amazing selection of fresh food available to you. Frozen, wild caught fish, with asparagus and a salad make a great meal that takes less than 20 minutes to put together. You do not have to be a chef to cook healthy meals that taste gourmet.

Instead of focusing on medicinal cures for cancer, diabetes, and heart disease, why don't we just clean up the diet and see what happens. I am sure this would have the most profound impact on the reduction of these deadly diseases. It is my wish that the American Heart Association and the American Cancer Association would spend their money here rather than on medications that cannot make up for poor eating habits.

Eat According to BLOOD TYPE

When you take an entire population and tell them to eat the same way, you are doing a great disservice to at least half of the population. We are not all the same. If you have the blood type O, eating red meat is extremely beneficial, while for A blood types, eating red meat is usually not appealing and symptoms of gastric distress are very common.

Dr. Peter D'Adamo is a naturopathic physician well known for his best selling books on the Blood Type Diet. His understanding of our dietary individuality has done more to help individuals suffering from inflammatory conditions and excess weight than anything else I have ever seen.

There has been no greater assistant to me when it comes to helping others with what ails them than initiating the Blood Type Diet. Years ago I did a paper that compared all the diets I could possibly find and research. I looked at the pros and cons of a large variety of diets. Are they healthy? Are you likely to rebound? Are you restricting too many essential nutrients or calories? Are you restricted to eating packaged diet foods?

When I looked at the piles of information I had in front of me, it seemed that the only "con" I could find about the Blood Type Diet was that it might make things difficult for a family of multiple blood types. Most individuals who incorporated this way of eating lost weight, decreased allergy symptoms, and had significant relief from inflammatory pain and digestive issues. If individuals were to incorporate this way of eating on a permanent basis, they would do more to prevent disease and illness than any supplement or medication ever could.

Blood typing is easy and inexpensive. It can even be done in your own home. A large majority of the population does not even know their blood type, including many doctors that I know. If I am doing a consultation, this is a very important piece of information that I need in order to help you make dietary choices that will potentially heal what ails you and add years to your life.

Mastication: CHEW YOUR FOOD!

You do it everyday, usually giving it very little thought. Some don't do it enough, which may lead to choking, and those that do it well will benefit. Mastication is the art of chewing.

Digestion begins in the mouth as we masticate or, more commonly stated, chew our food. It is here that the food is mixed with saliva, which contains enzymes. The more you chew your food, the more you give your body a digestive head start.

No one is guiltier than yours truly when it comes to inhaling food. I love to eat, and fortunately, love healthy wholesome foods. Where I need some work is in slowing down long enough to enjoy each and every bite, and not swallowing pieces of food practically in their whole food form. I'll explain why this is so important.

Chewing at least 25 times per mouthful will dramatically improve the digestive ability of your body. When food is kept in the mouth, the taste on the tongue prompts the release of the hormones, digestive enzymes, and gastric juices that begin to soften and liquefy the food in order to prepare for the passage to the stomach.

Well-chewed food travels easily from mouth to stomach. Poorly chewed food tends to be dryer and has difficulty making its way to the stomach. Chewing thoroughly is very important when it come to your health. Well-chewed food has more surface area for the gastric juices and enzymes to work in your stomach. At the same time, your stomach is churning until most of the digested food is the consistency of a paste called chyme. Much of your body's energy is needed to perform this task. The better you chew, the less energy is required for this task, leaving your body free for other important duties. Chewing well also decreases the likelihood that it will spend a longer time in the stomach causing fermentation, gas, and burping, and even heartburn.

Masticating, or chewing, can be thought of as a type of juicing. Nutrients are distributed much more rapidly to the cells where they are needed. As an added bonus, chewing also stimulates the parotid glands, which can give your immune system a boost.

For some, including myself, this may take a bit of practice. Eating on the go is not conducive to digesting properly and every effort should be make to avoid this situation. For the first week or so make a conscious effort to chew your food 20-25 times before swallowing. Most of you will have to actually count, but after a while it will become habit. You will soon come to know what a well-chewed carrot feels like in the mouth and will not likely swallow the large pieces you once did.

The art of mastication is the cheapest and easiest way of improving your digestive health. If you make chewing a priority and daily practice, you may find that over time you will require fewer digestive aids and even less medication.

Chapter 4

Common Causes of Your Backed-Up Plumbing

Ignoring Nature's Call for Elimination

The inappropriate timing of nature's call to move your bowels is what causes many of us to start heading down the path toward a constipated life. Many individuals, especially women, will not use the work place bathroom and will only go at home. This holding problem most likely originated in the early school years. Missing your window of "poopertunity" initiates the downward spiral to a life of constipation.

I'll refresh you on the anatomy of this situation. First of all, we must remember that one of the main functions of the large intestine is to absorb water. The longer your poop remains in there, the harder it becomes. The harder your waste becomes, the harder it is to pass through when you decide to finally go. Many lose the urge all together, and amazingly, can go a few days before the urge strikes again. I really don't know how some people just don't blow up.

Over time, the lower part of the colon becomes over-distended or stretched out to accommodate your unwillingness to "go". Every once in a while you'll tend to have that great bowel movement and feel more energetic and light again for a few days. Most likely, the bowel movement was painful, large and may have caused some bleeding. Did you need the plunger? Once empty, it will be days before you go again and the vicious cycle continues.

Hemorrhoids are a common complication of this scenario. This over-distended colon causes pelvic congestion that makes blood-flow difficult in this area. This causes your veins to become distended (like your colon) and hemorrhoids become part of your world.

The longer this state of affairs is allowed to continue, the more difficult it is to reverse. Muscle tone is lost, and even after a great bowel movement you have all this room to refill over the next few days. Daily or twice daily bowel movements are almost impossible without the help of stimulants, which can be very habit forming and only contribute to the lack of tone in the bowel.

Anatomically Incorrect

Based on what I've seen in practice, I would estimate that at least 10 to 15 percent of the population is anatomically incorrect. Meaning that those pretty pictures of a "normal" colon is the case for some, but not for all. These individuals come in for help with constipation and they usually have had these issues all of their life.

Unfortunately these individuals will struggle with constipation issues that typically span their lifetime. For them, colon hydrotherapy is a valuable tool for maintaining health. The challenge is that they usually find supplements that work well for them, but the benefits and better bowel movements are short-lived. Eventually the product or supplement stops working for them. The best advice I can give is to keep the colon hydrotherapy appointments regular. The toolbox that has accumulated over the years full of remedies that once worked will come in handy. Keep it close, and switch things up often—this is key. This will usually keep you out of harms way.

I have already told you about Anne and her near death experience. I believe Anne had suffered from an anatomically incorrect colon. This predisposed her to a life full of unexplained constipation.

Sometimes it is the lack of abdominal muscle or failure to heal the abdominal muscle wall after surgery or pregnancy that is the problem. This is a fairly common condition that most physicians and their patients rarely consider to be a factor in difficulty down the road. Diastasis recti, also known as, "mommy belly," is a common medical condition in which the tissues of the abdomen, particularly the abdominal muscles, are stretched apart and separated. It occurs most often as a result of pregnancy.

Here is the story of Debbie, who actually found her own "cure" once we were able to determine what the problem was. Debbie is a beautiful mom in her mid-forties with a lean body and not an ounce of fat, and she worked hard for that. She did however have this mini-Buddha belly that she obsessed over, which just seemed out of place on someone so physically fit. Here is her "anatomically incorrect" story in her own words:

My story begins around 1995. After 3 years of trying to get pregnant (had fertility tests, took Clomid) I had a laparoscopy. The doctor mentioned that I had excessive scar tissue and asked if I had ever had an infection or other complications growing up. I didn't as far as I knew; I have an extremely high tolerance for pain/discomfort so if there was anything wrong I probably wouldn't have realized it anyway.

We actually gave up trying and that's when I got pregnant with daughter #1 at the age of 33, then had daughter #2 at the age of 35. I always had a slim, athletic build, never dieted in my life, never really worked out. I was never "regular" but didn't give it much thought; it was 'normal' to me.

After kids, things went downhill. When my kids were about 5 and 4, respectively, I was starting to feel anxious, frustrated beyond belief, etc. I've always worked full-time and I was feeling overwhelmed: carting kids to/from school, to/from the sitter, keeping up with work/home/husband, dealing with mommy-guilt, etc. I was sitting at my desk at work one day, and felt like my heart was racing, like I was moving 60 mph but I was sitting still.

I don't consider myself stressed but I've always heard that stress can do strange things to you without you even realizing it. My PCP (primary care physician) had been suggesting for months prior that I take celexa but I refused because I'm not a medicine taker. I wasn't interested in masking the symptoms of whatever it was that was wrong, I was bent on finding the root cause and fixing it.

Against my better judgment and since I honestly felt like I was headed for a breakdown at this point, I ended up taking the celexa. I was told that it'd take about 2 weeks for it to get into my system and work to where I noticed a difference. Well, after a couple days, I knew it was working.

I recall sitting on the couch in the living room one day with a cup of tea watching my girls put up window clings for whatever holiday happened to be coming up. They were having fun helping Mommy "decorate", and the clings were on the window in nothing close to a nice orderly pattern; they were overlapping, multiple ones clumped in one corner, a couple on top of each other, it was a mess. And you know what? I didn't care! My normal Type A tendencies were so muted by this "medicine" that I didn't care that my window looked like you-know-what. And, I didn't fix it, either. I left it just like that thru that holiday.

Now, maybe some would think that that's not a big deal, so what that the window looked like that. And they'd be right...I loved that my girls were having fun however, knowing and feeling that my "self" was so altered so as to not even have had the desire to discreetly rearrange the clings when they went to bed, for example, was enough to scare me so that I threw the pills away and never took them again. Never mind that you aren't supposed to abruptly stop taking them, I didn't want anything to do with them anymore.

So, at that point I was about 40 and decided to get serious about health & fitness. Even though I was spending at least 4-5 days at the gym, working with a personal trainer, watching what I ate, etc., I was still not "regular" and, the most frustrating of all, I could not get rid of my pouchy belly no matter what I did. I felt bloated and gassy all the time, would get what I assumed were gas pains so bad they would stop me in my tracks until the episode passed. I was still fitting into my usual clothes but I felt (and felt that I looked like) a beached whale. It was awful.

I saw my primary physician again, had blood work that revealed that I have Hashimoto's

Free Yourself from a **CONSTIPATED** *Life*

Disease but that was about it, otherwise perfectly healthy. Autoimmune issues run in my family—and, from what I understand, autoimmune diseases are rampant in WNY (Western New York). My siblings suffer from such ailments as Type I diabetes, rheumatoid arthritis, fibromyalgia, Reynaud's disease, limited scleroderma, and a myriad of other things. I'm the oldest of 5 and, thankfully, have none of these. I'm tested once a year to ensure that the Hashimoto's hasn't developed into anything further. I asked about the irregularity and pouchy belly and was told to eat more whole wheat, fiber, etc.

I'm open to supplements, vitamins, herbs, etc. but prefer to avoid taking medicine for something unless absolutely necessary. I started using Metamucil—totally gross and I could barely drink it. But I did. Nothing. No results. I tried tweaking the dosage, used less, then more. Got frustrated after weeks of using it to no avail and gave up. So, I took to the Internet and came across a product for a cleanse. I read all the information on the website and read the testimonials; it sounded like just what I was looking for!

I ordered the regimen, which consisted of a fiber mix (tasted good, actually), probiotics, a multivitamin, and senna tea. While I never got results like those depicted on the website, I felt that the program was working. I was

*more regular, less bloated, I felt "lighter". I
continued working out and watching what I
was eating but still, I knew I wasn't 100%.*

*I used the products for about four years and
did a 90-day cleanse each of those years. In
the fourth year, I did two cleanses because I
was starting to feel like I was regressing
somehow. Although my symptoms were
alleviated, they weren't completely gone and
they were starting now to come back with a
vengeance. I couldn't figure out why. I used
the senna tea to excess; the directions said to
steep the tea for no more than ten minutes.
Well, I was getting absolutely no results so I
started leaving the tea bag in the cup the
whole time I was drinking it! Not good
apparently because liver damage could
result. Great...I'm trying to fix myself and
was potentially causing more harm. Nothing
happened, thank goodness, but needless to
say I stopped using the senna.*

*OK, so I have all these things going on at
this point: crazy schedule (who's isn't?!),
irregularity, bloating, and now my periods
are getting screwy and libido is rapidly
declining. I thought the 40's are supposed to
be a fabulous time for women?! To that I
say HAH! Not the case for me.*

*So back to the PCP and GYN I go. I mention
all the issues, that fiber isn't working, belly*

88

is distended, I feel bloated, etc. Now, don't get me wrong, I really like my doctors otherwise I wouldn't be a patient of theirs, and I go to women purposely because I don't feel that a man can possibly "get" the things that women go through, whether it be mentally, physically, whatever. But, I was told that what I was experiencing was part of life, I was over 40 after all. I may be in peri-menopause, perfectly normal.

Add that to the list of "issues"! And. with that comes a whole new set of things to deal with—the most disturbing being that my libido was not only declining, it had become almost non-existent. At some point during one of my GYN visits, my doctor suggested I contact Cathi Stack at Journey II Health. I took the information and actually emailed Cathi a couple times for some information but never made an appointment to follow up.

The online products/cleanse that I had been using were working until just around the time of this particular GYN appointment, and my trainer had mentioned something called the Blood Type Diet that I was also looking into. Thus, I didn't pursue an appointment at Journey II Health at this point (in hindsight, baaaad decision).

Through all of this, I was continuing to work out, watch what I ate, and had become officially obsessed with my abdomen and how to fix it. No matter where I went, I focused on other womens' abs (How are her abs so flat and mine aren't? What am I doing wrong? What IS this thing that won't go away?).

My distended abdomen was on my mind every second of every day. The PCP mentioned that I had an umbilical hernia, most likely caused by my pregnancies. She said that there really was no hurry to get it fixed, I wasn't feeling any pain, etc. so, I didn't pursue surgery.

This whole process has been an approximate 8-year quest to determine what was "wrong" with me, my belly to be specific. I had been working out (circuit training, Pilates, Body Pump) & walking religiously, able to build great looking arms, legs...mid-section always looked distended, like a beach ball. I could not figure out why as I've always had a thin athletic build, no reason that I still shouldn't, right?

I modified my diet, did more crunches, etc. to no avail. My belly button looked like it had an eyelid that was half closed. Also, if I bent or moved the wrong way, it felt like a little fist would pop out from under my right rib and I had to push it back in...freaked me out whenever it happened. I used to joke that one of my organs was popping out (the irony sets in later).

I finally had the umbilical hernia repaired in May 2010, hoping that that would improve the appearance of the belly button and the beach ball...no luck.

I'm embarrassed to admit it, but I actually did nine treatments of Zerona, the laser treatment to remove fat by targeting specific areas (there was a Groupon or Seize the Deal for the procedure but it was still way expensive). Guess what? Total waste of money because, in my case, it wasn't a fat issue. I didn't know this at the time, of course, but read on.

I saw a plastic surgeon twice, considering a tummy tuck. My obsession with my abdomen had literally consumed my every waking moment, I felt I was at the end of my rope, thinking there was nothing else for me to do. Ultimately, I couldn't bring myself to spend that kind of money, go thru the recovery process (no patience to be down that long), or have the unsightly scar from hip to hip.

Fast forward to October of 2011. I finally made an appointment with Cathi. Our first meeting lasted about an hour or so and she really listened to me. She got what I was saying. Finally! I left feeling encouraged that I was on the road to recovery. She suggested some supplements to balance the hormones. She also is the only other one, besides my trainer that I know of, that is familiar with the Blood Type Diet.

I'm A+ and I learned that wheat is not my friend. I also discovered that I'm sensitive to gluten. I can tell when I've eaten too many of the crap foods because the rash on the insides of my elbows will make its appearance. It itches like crazy but goes away when I stop eating the junk and eat more of what I should.

At my fourth colonic with her, I was lamenting about my belly (again). Cathi is also a midwife and happens to be a friend of my good friend who is a labor & delivery RN. She's feeling around my belly and mentioned that my muscles felt separated & mushy. Good, I wasn't the only one who thought so, so maybe I wasn't crazy after all.

I got home after that appointment and was relaying the experience to my friend, the L&D nurse. Within minutes, she had googled diastasis recti. I heard trumpets from the heavens! For the next 2 days, I was searching everything I could find on this, read that umbilical hernias are a result of a diastasis, the abs actually are separated, and (holy cow), it probably was an organ popping out from under my rib when I bent/moved the wrong way! I discovered a program to fix the condition and am currently pursuing becoming licensed so that I can teach it to others so that they can heal as well. (The Tupler Technique was developed by Julie Tupler, RN.)

I had spent eight years of my life thinking I was not able to get in shape, crazy, or just plain vain. I just couldn't (and wouldn't) buy into the notion that this puffy belly was something I had to deal with because I was a woman, a mom, over 45, blah, blah, blah.

Cathi was the catalyst to me finding this program to fix the belly thing and, as a result of that and in combination with the supplements and colonics, I've been able to heal my anatomy. I no longer feel bloated, my belly is not distended—in fact, I've lost four inches off my waist! I'm more regular than I've ever been in my life, and, I no longer have to pee every 10 minutes (or so it seemed)!

Cathi is genuinely concerned about the health and wellness of others and has a gift to heal what ails a body. I am so thankful that I know her and will continue to seek her guidance and healing. I am also firm believer in fate; I was meant to meet Cathi

*and she was meant to "fix" me. I told her
when we first met that I was not textbook
and that I would be her "project". I think I
fulfilled that prediction.*

Stressed Out & Controlling

Women seem to be more prone to constipation during
times of stress. Two thoughts come to my mind:
  1) They can't let their shit go.
  2) By holding on (literally, to their shit) they think
     they have control.
There is a fine line between being in control of your life
and being a "control freak", and I teeter that line more
than I'd like to admit. For the most part, I'm happy to say
that I'm not a control freak, no matter what my husband
might say!

People having a balanced sense of control of their
life definitely understand that the universe can and will
throw curve balls at the most inopportune time. They may
not like it, but they will adjust to whatever the
circumstance is and continue to move on. The control
freak is likely to have a meltdown, need years of therapy,
or maybe even medications for anxiety and depression.
Many have a martyr-like disposition.

Now, it is only natural to want to be in control of
your own life, but when you feel you have to have control
of everybody else's lives, you have a problem. These are
the key aspects of a "control freak". They have a driving
need to create your agenda; they insist on controlling all
their interactions with you; basically, they have to run the
show and call the shots—OR ELSE.

94

It has been found that the main need to control is driven by anxiety, though a control freak would never recognize this; even if they did, they would deny it. At work, they worry about failure. In their relationships, they dread that they will not have their needs met, or that they will not be good enough. In order to keep this anxiety from overwhelming them, they feel the only way to avoid feeling those emotions is to control the people or things around them. They have a harder time than most normal people when it comes to negotiation or compromise, because it would mean they would have to give up some of their control, and it would also implicate that they are not perfect. Control freaks H-A-T-E imperfection. If by now you can't tell or don't already know, this can make life difficult; whether you are working with them, living with them, or just plain stuck in a circle involving them.

The reason most of us don't like control freaks is because they always give off the impression that we're incompetent, or cannot be trusted. I'm not saying they don't act out of love or in your best interest; they often do, but the anxiety and fear of a potential "out of control" situation can be toxic to any environment where they are involved.

We all come to this life with gifts on board for a reason, a lesson, and even a purpose. It is difficult to believe that anyone's purpose is to control someone else. For a time, raising children is all consuming and rewarding—but it doesn't last forever and isn't supposed to. Marriage, relationships, and partnerships of respect should not be controlling, but provide a venue for mutual growth. If you truly love someone, then wouldn't you love to watch him or her evolve into his or her full potential? The control freak would probably want to dictate what that potential should be. Many try to control their loved ones for fear of losing them. People tire of being controlled and such relationships suffer and potentially end. Being controlled often leads to someone "flying the coop". They feel they are suffocating and human instinct will lead to "fight or flight". Rest assured, the controlled party does finally leave. The more you try to control or resist change, the more you are doomed to the reality that change IS the one guarantee in life. Stress and potential illness may occur within the body of those who try to control that which they ultimately cannot.

Having total control of anything in life is an illusion. In any given moment things can change—and that's just the way it is. Living in a "go with the flow" attitude, will unfold the benefits of stress-free living. This should also have a go-with-the-flow effect on your colon. The weight that will be lifted from your shoulders will add years to your life. People will enjoy your company rather than avoid you. Life becomes easier and you begin to enjoy the "priceless" moments that you would normally miss attempting to be in control.

You are not in control of anyone but your own destiny, so you must learn to let "it" go and enjoy the ride. This thought pattern has an amazing way of correlating with more frequent bowel movements.

Louise Hay, famous author and publisher, defines a probable cause of constipation to be, "Refusing to release old ideas, stuck in the past. Sometimes stinginess." The new thought pattern that should take place, according to Louise is, "As I release the past, the new and fresh and vital enter, I allow life to flow through me." Another helpful thought pattern would be, "I freely and easily release the old, and joyously welcome the new."

Believe it or not, the above paragraph when put into play, actually helps individuals release thought patterns that may be a contributing factor to their constipated ways.

Medication Maladies

I distinctly remember way back in nursing school that many side effects were the same for many medications. We had to memorize the medications, doses, generic names, contraindications, what they were used for and all of the possible side effects. How is one to remember all of this? I cannot tell you how many index cards were made up in order to remember these details. Then one day I had a revelation. If, when tested on most medications, I listed nausea, vomiting, headache, diarrhea and constipation, I would never be marked incorrect.

That being said, medications are a very common cause and contributing factor to constipation in many individuals. Pain medications are at the top of the list.

Narcotics are prescribed to help with pain. Unfortunately, many people stay on them longer than needed with no plans to reduce or wean the dose down. This sets many up for addictions and failure to work through therapies that will improve their situation. I know many individuals who have become addicted to pain medications and prefer to stay there, as it is the easier option. This is a sad state of affairs.

Narcotic and opiates affect bowel function in a variety of ways, the first of which is by delaying gastric emptying. Pain medications delay transit time by affecting normal tone and contractility of the small and large intestine. Besides this, the sensation numbing effect of these medications cause the individual to overlook the urge to have a bowel movement, and the limited or restricted mobility following surgery does not help either.

Now I am not saying that you should not take pain medications if you have just had surgery or an injury that requires them—just make sure someone is paying attention to your bowel health. Taking stool softeners and/or laxatives will come in handy during this time. I have seen many individuals who remember constipation in their postoperative period to be the pain they remember most.

Many individuals are placed on diuretics for high blood pressure, fluid retention, or both. Diuretics increase water elimination via the kidneys, making less water available to the colon. Stool becomes harder and more difficult to pass.

I have recently seen many individuals placed on medications for an overactive bladder, or better described as the urge to go even when your bladder is not full. Dry mouth and constipation are two of the more common side effects of these drugs.

Antidepressants, blood pressure medications, anticonvulsants and even iron supplements are responsible for constipation among the many individuals taking them.

Please do not stop taking these medications if they were prescribed to you. This needs to be discussed with your doctor. Be aware of the possibility of constipation and the need to proactively prevent it.

Laxative abuse may ultimately be responsible for constipation. The forced stimulation of the colon over long periods of time renders the colon useless and unable to function on its own. I have actually had the personal experience of seeing a colon during surgery that was obviously suffering from the effects of years of abuse. If I did not know that the patient was alive, I would have bet I was looking at a colon of a corpse. It was very pale and looked lifeless. The girl was only in her mid-twenties. This is a common finding in those with eating disorders and laxative abuse.

Scar Tissue & Adhesions Have You in a Bind?

Any type of abdominal surgery can be a set up for constipation in the future, as healing tissue has a way of making your insides stick together. The more surgery you have, the more likely you are to have adhesions. Endometriosis causes adhesions as well.

Adhesions develop as the body attempts to heal itself from injury or surgery. Even radiation can cause adhesions. A surgery complicated by infection will likely have more adhesions than one that heals without difficulty.

While the injured or surgical site is healing, the cells within the body cannot differentiate between one organ and another. Have you ever cut yourself and noticed that even when the bleeding stops, there is a clear drainage that follows? This is serous fluid and it tends to be sticky as it dries. Well, simply put, if this is going on the inside of your body, scar tissue will form and may connect two surfaces that were not supposed to be connected.

Adhesions typically begin to form within a few days after surgery, but may not show symptoms for months and even years. Just like your arteries and other organs, they may become hardened as we age from a combination of poor diet and sedentary ways. This may lead to difficult passage through the intestines, causing sluggish bowels and in the worst case, a blockage. Typically, there are no major complications with adhesion formation—so don't worry. Adhesions will occur in about 90 percent of all people who undergo abdominal or pelvic surgery. Occasionally some individuals may suffer from pulling or pinching sensations as their body heals.

In about 10 percent of my clientele, constipation was never an issue until there had been an abdominal event or surgery that precipitated their symptoms.

Here is another story of how a poor diet, extreme anxiety or intensity, and surgical complications could negatively impact your life. Coach has become one of my favorite clients. I will tell you honestly that he was one of the more challenging personalities I have ever had to work with. I never thought I would look forward to his visits—we laugh about this now.

This is Coach McNally's story in his own words:

My name is Jim McNally. I am a retired NFL football coach. I coached 15 years in college and 30 years in the NFL. I moved my family 10 times and had 9 jobs. My entire working career was filled with constant stress. The NFL is short for "no fun league" or "not for long." It's win or else.

During my career I ate anything and everything. It was normal to eat a whole large pizza with everything on it and drink 5-

6 diet cokes a day. I had no idea about healthy eating, alkaline diets, or food combination.

I never had unusually high cholesterol and my blood tests generally were normal. When I retired in 2008 from the Buffalo Bills I had pains in my stomach, belching, etc. It seems that after years of unhealthy eating, pouring aspartame down my gut, (diet cokes) and constant stress that acid erosion developed in my esophagus, I was diagnosed with "Barretts Syndrome," which is a precancerous condition. I went on a proton pump inhibitor called Zegerid to rid the acid in my stomach.

In 2008 I established my own LLC, consulting all over the country doing football clinics, seminars, private sessions at high schools, colleges, professional teams, and camps. I created my own website, selling DVD's and advertising my skills as a retired football coaching consultant, majoring in offensive line play.

In the summer of 2010 I was at a high school in Grand Rapids, MI. After tutoring players and coaches I returned to my hotel and felt sick. At 2:00am I had awful stomach pains and called 911. An ambulance came and took me to a hospital in Grand Rapids. They took two cat scans, one with dye and one without. The one with dye showed I had a problem with my appendix. They did not operate on me until 8:30pm. My appendix had burst.

After stitching me up and giving me antibiotics and pain meds, I left the hospital in Michigan and flew home to Buffalo the next day. They allowed me to leave because I was able to urinate on my own.

After returning to Buffalo, I was as sick as a dog. Cramping, couldn't poop, and was scared. I called a top man in the radiology department at a local Buffalo hospital and checked in the following day.

At the hospital in Buffalo they took a cat scan and saw I had two major abscesses and a bowel blockage. My surgeon said we need to open you up and clean you out, as I was in serious condition. When your appendix bursts, the poison within coats your insides and forms scar tissue. The poisons burning my organs along with a major seven-inch incision added to the internal scarring.

After a month in and out of the hospital, on antibiotics, losing 25 lbs, I was on the long road to recovery. I could not poop very well since my stomach had shut down while I was healing, as it takes time to come alive.

After eating I would feel full and lots of pain. The food would expand my colon and hit the scar tissue and wow—"pain pain pain."

I ran into a friend who sent me to my first angel. This friend says I will fix you up with "Tom." Tom is an anatomical engineer who digs out scar tissue all over your body. He got into my stomach with deep massage treatments and helped soften the scar tissue.

All the time I thought I was constipated as all the pain, healing, stress on my stomach and worry made my bowel movements poor and infrequent. I was so stressed and positive that I was constipated that I took laxatives and became dependent on them. All this time I wasn't really constipated, just the scar tissue created so much pain, and as I overstressed I created my own anxiety and constipation.

Tom said, " You need to see Cathi". This was my next angel. Cathi said she couldn't give me a colonic for nine months or so because of the recent surgery but she could help me with recommendations on diet and supplements.

Cathi put me on digestive enzymes, probiotics, Vitamin D-3, magnesium, Cape Aloe, and helped me get my bathroom habits normal again. She gave me the proper diet corresponding with my blood type and guaranteed me that I would be all right.

After nine months I had my first colonic with Cathi and have been going to her once a month for over a year. She has changed my life.

On another matter, I was on that proton pump inhibitor to take the acid out of my stomach to help heal my "Barrett's Syndrome" which was discussed earlier. After two years on the pill, I had an endoscopy, where they took a biopsy of my esophagus and the cells were healing.

The proton pump inhibitors can create damage to your system when taken over a long period of time, leading to osteoporosis and malnutrition. I tried to stop the pill abruptly, but couldn't do it as my body was so used to the drug that my acid reflux symptoms were too great to stop the medication.

Cathi gave me a plan to wean myself off the drug by alternating a lesser degree of the pill, then to Zantac, and then to total avoidance of the drug. She was a Godsend.

Her soothing demeanor, her knowledge of colon health, and the healing of other body parts along with her being an expert on the top supplements used for a healthy life make her the expert she is.

Stress was a big part of my problem. I am type A and actually "make coffee nervous." Cathi identified that my adrenal glands were so fired up and off the charts that she put me on a supplement that managed cortisol levels, which slows your adrenal glands "fight mechanism" down and I was able to sleep better at night and relax more than ever.

Cathi also helped me with supplements for parasites as the pains I had after surgery may have been caused by them. When your stomach shuts down the parasites may have congregated at the healing sits also causing constipation. After two doses of Cathi's parasite killers I was moving my bowels daily.

For almost six months I would email Cathi almost daily complaining of one thing after another. She put up with a lot of my worries and calmed me down when I was about to go crazy.

After have a colonic with Cathi, I feel light, free, with no anxiety. The colonic rids your body of waste stuck in your colon that puts you in a sluggish, bloated and unhappy mood.

I wouldn't go without my monthly colonic and my supplements. Cathi saved my life and my association with her took my stress level from off the charts to normal.

She is truly an angel sent to me. When she arrived I tapped her for every bit of her knowledge and more. More than a colon manager, she is a lifesaver of the greatest magnitude.

Body Mechanics

You probably have not given the topic of body mechanics much thought, but it should be considered. Mother nature intended for us to eliminate in the squatting position. Even in childbirth, this is the position that many women would naturally choose to deliver their babies.

Complications such as constipation are a result of the anatomical position that the toilet puts us in. By avoiding the squatting position, we predispose ourselves to hemorrhoids, hernias and incomplete emptying of the colon.

The toilet first originated in England somewhere around 1850. Although many believe that Thomas Crapper invented the toilet, the original design came from Alexander Cumming. Thomas Crapper did actually come to patent many versions of the toilet and some poop advocates might accuse him of a crappy job.

Many places in the world today still have just a

hole in the floor for toilets. People who use these will rarely suffer from constipation or hemorrhoids. Infection rates are low as well.

So now what? Should your rip your toilet out leaving a hole in the floor to defecate in? I would hope not. An easy remedy to the situation would be to add a footstool to your bathroom that is within reach of the toilet. While sitting on the toilet, place your feet on the stool and pull them close to the body. This will assist your body in finding that natural squatting position is has been longing for.

At Journey II Health, we keep a stool in the bathroom so that following a colon hydrotherapy session you may optimize the evacuation of your colon. This tip sounds so very simple but is likely to have profound benefits in your quest to eliminate constipation.

Chapter 5

Supplements & Foods: Friends With Benefits

B ecause the FDA (Food and Drug Administration) is not likely to spend millions of dollars to prove that natural remedies or foods are safe in the prevention or resolution of constipation, most of what I say here is based on personal experience and is unlikely to be FDA approved, ever. So in this section I can only say, " none of these therapies are FDA approved to relieve you of constipation." You be the judge.

The Truth About FIBER

Most constipated individuals are told they need to take fiber supplements. This may be the worst advice anyone could ever give to someone who is already backed up. Fiber is a bulking agent that will actually make the constipated individual even more uncomfortable, at least until the problem is resolved. For the "unconstipated" individual, fiber is a great way to keep things moving and prevent complications of constipation.

There are two types of fiber—soluble fiber and insoluble fiber. Insoluble fiber does not absorb water, whereas soluble fiber does. Most over the counter fiber products are composed of soluble fiber. Some fiber products tend to ferment in the colon, making things a bit uncomfortable for many individuals.

The best way to describe fiber is to imagine that it is the skeleton of a plant. Like a straw broom, it sweeps the lining of our colon clean, absorbs excess fluids, and quickly exits the body, taking toxic residue with it.

Those suffering with chronic diarrhea would have great results from taking fiber, as it would slow them down and bulk them up. Why then, do most medical and health-conscious professionals seem to be giving such poor advice? If the individual ate a diet high in fiber, they wouldn't be in this predicament in the first place.

When "Anatomy and Physiology" is taught in school, it only makes sense to assume that fiber would benefit the colon. So for a profession that does not correlate food with health, I can see why this advice is given.

The sad fact of the matter is, if we all ate a healthy diet, (most individuals don't know what that is), we would not need laxatives and softening agents. Fiber would keep us out of trouble.

Fruits, vegetables, nuts and whole grains are the BEST sources of fiber. Many of my patients barely get one or two servings in a day when I initially consult with them.

Avocados contain approximately 11 grams of fiber and artichokes contain 10 grams. The current recommendation for fiber consumption is 35 grams per day. I feel this should be the bare minimum and you should strive for much more. Raspberries, blackberries and lentils contain 9 grams of fiber per cup. These are just a few examples of great food sources for fiber. Food is always your best source of fiber. Although both have benefits, chia seeds are higher in fiber than flaxseed. Three tablespoons of chia seeds contain 15 grams of fiber, while three tablespoons of flaxseed contain 9 grams of fiber.

If you are already suffering from backed-up plumbing, be very wary of man-made products boasting loads of fiber. This may backfire on you.

Get things moving first and then begin to incorporate a diet high in natural fiber.

Digestive Enzymes

Anyone with digestive difficulty should pay attention and consider incorporating digestive enzymes into their daily supplement regime.

From a nutritional standpoint, most of the digestive misery that many suffer from could have been avoided if only enzymes were understood. A diet that consists mostly of cooked and processed foods will ultimately suffer from the effects of enzyme depletion.

Enzymes are tiny protein molecules found in the foods we eat. They are responsible and necessary for the breakdown of foods into absorbable nutrients. Enzymes provide us the life force energy that keeps our bodies functioning optimally.

Research shows that if your food is not digested properly, the side effects range from bloating, lactose intolerance, stomach discomfort, gas, indigestion, heartburn, acid reflux, allergies, skin problems, some kinds of cancer, fatigue and premature aging. Products such as antacids and acid blockers only stop digestion and interfere with nutrient absorption. What is the percentage of raw foods you consume daily? If you consume less than 40 percent of your daily food in the raw form, you are likely to be suffering in an enzyme deficient state. If you do not tolerate raw foods, the condition of enzyme deficiency is well established and something should be done.

Unfortunately, most individuals consume their food cooked. Enzymes are destroyed at temperatures of 118 degrees and above. Anytime you cook, microwave, fry, bake, or grill your food; consider it enzyme deficient.

So now you ask yourself, "How bad is this anyway?" Fortunately our bodies were built with a backup supply of digestive enzymes for us to borrow, but the supply is limited. So depending on your diet; the indigestion, heartburn, IBS and other maladies will show up earlier or later in life.

The more enzyme deficient you become, the harder your body has to work. Eating cooked and processed food will most probably lead to frequent sickness, premature aging and other biological inconveniences. By taking digestive enzymes with meals, you are providing your body with the ability to properly break down your foods. This is extremely helpful to those suffering with digestive issues as well as allergies. The inconvenience of taking them with meals is soon forgotten as many individuals begin to notice improvements within a week or so. Situational supplementation can help you as well. I am Italian and I love macaroni, or as most would call it, pasta.

Because of my O blood type, pasta is an inflammatory food for me, which is easily demonstrated in the two to three inches that magically appear around my waistline within an hour or two. If I know I will be eating pasta, digestive enzymes will prevent some of the body drama and disfigurement.

There are many different types of digestive enzymes on the market. You should look for a product containing a multiple selection of plant enzymes. For example; protease digests protein, amylase digests sugars, lipase digests fats, and so on. You need a stabilized formula that will survive a hostile gut, as well as one that contains chelated minerals for optimal performance. Many high quality enzymes will also contain probiotics, which becomes our next topic.

Probiotics

Although I consider them essential for health, there is quite a bit of confusion on the topic of probiotics, also known as "healthy bacteria". On this, I'd like to shed some light. First understand that "pro" means "for" and "biotic" means "life". Therefore, probiotic = for life.

Probiotics are finally being understood for their extreme importance in supporting intestinal health and immune system strength. Stomach upset, fatigue, frequent colds and flus, and sensitivity to milk and dairy products are some of the signs that your friendly bacteria need to be replenished. As I have said earlier, 80 percent of your immune system lies within the gut.

Antibiotics (against life) kill not only the bad bacteria (which can be life-saving at times), but also kill the friendly bacteria that we need for health and

113

wellbeing. Unfortunately, even if we haven't taken prescription antibiotics we are still regularly exposed to them. Since half of the antibiotics produced each year are fed to animals, we take in antibiotics every time we eat meat or dairy products. If that is not enough, the body's friendly bacterium is depleted by many other factors including stress, carbonation, laxatives and even the natural aging process.

The human body is made up of an estimated 100 trillion bacterial cells from at least 500 species, not including viruses and fungi. These bacteria (probiotics) are referred to as "friendly" bacteria and are responsible for several important biological functions. Some of these functions include assisting in digestion, keeping other harmful bacteria at bay, and stimulating the immune system. A healthy "GUT" is essential for a healthy immune system. Adults and children, including infants, would all benefit from the use of probiotics on a regular basis. The need for antibiotics would be greatly reduced, and the hopeful reduction of resistant strains of bacteria would likely occur.

The Standard American Diet (SAD) that consists of mostly processed and refined foods contributes to an unhealthy environment consisting of an overgrowth of yeast (Candida) and unfriendly bacteria. Those who eat commonly advertised yogurts for the purpose of adding friendly bacteria would have to eat approximately two gallons per day to get what a good supplement would offer. Not only that, but most advertised yogurts are loaded with artificial flavors, sweeteners and chemical processing—YUK!

Thankfully, many doctors are not so quick to prescribe unnecessary antibiotics, as they are aware this has definitely contributed to the formation of "superbugs" or resistant strains of bacteria that can be deadly to us. Probiotics would benefit every person at any age. Once a day dosing makes it easy and convenient. If you notice a gurgling, bloated feeling after taking them, it may suggest yeast or Candida overgrowth, which means you need them all the more. Many people also suffer skin rashes and infections that could have been avoided had they been taking probiotics. Wounds heal faster and the risk for infection is greatly reduced.

Unfortunately not all probiotics are the same. I see many taking acidophilus, which is only one of the many strains we need. Therefore, it is not very effective as a single remedy. A stabilized, multi-strain formula works best. There are some excellent products out there that do not require refrigeration, as well as some that do. Quality matters, as it is very important that the healthy bacteria be stable enough to survive the long drive through the intestinal tract.

Anyone suffering from IBS, chronic constipation, diverticulosis, diverticulitis, colitis, frequent yeast or Candida issues, or an immune system that is less than adequate would benefit from daily supplementation.

I highly recommend probiotics following ANY antibiotic treatment. Sadly, this is rarely recommended. Antibiotics can be life saving in some situations, but they also kill the friendly bacteria. We need to replace the good bacteria very quickly in order to maximize a rapid return to health and healing, and to prevent a recurrence of illness.

Cape Aloe

More individuals are familiar with the liquid aloe supplements derived from the aloe plant than capsules made from the leaf. Liquid aloe is very beneficial when soothing symptoms in the upper digestive tract, and I recommend it often.

The aloe I will refer to for the purpose of constipation relief is Cape Aloe or aloe ferox. Cape Aloe is one of the most effective softening agents I have come to know. It has helped the majority of my constipated clientele and is one of our best sellers. It is very gentle and unlike some other herbal remedies, does not cause cramping or uncomfortable blowouts. Dosing varies per individual and daily supplementation is not the goal. Initially, daily supplementation may be necessary to establish bowel movements once or twice daily. Usage two to three times weekly in order to keep things moving is the desired goal.

You'd be wise to let this become one of your dearest travel companions, as many individuals often find themselves constipated when they travel. Even those who do not suffer from constipation are sure to improve the experience of their travel companions by having this handy. Our "Poop Kit" at Journey II Health contains Cape Aloe and deodorizing poop drops, which help make even the shyest bathroom user much more confident without the embarrassment of odor. Cape Aloe is safe and I have even recommended it to pregnant moms with great results. Being constipated is unsafe!

Magnesium

The mineral magnesium is an extremely under utilized supplement that has far more benefit in the human body than the overly used calcium. Magnesium deficiency is one of the most common causes of constipation and is frequently overlooked. Other signs of deficiency include muscle cramps, restless leg, heart palpitations and maybe even high blood pressure.

The laxative effect of magnesium is most likely the result of two different mechanisms. Magnesium is a muscle relaxer, and the colon and small intestines are muscles. Magnesium will help to establish peristalsis, which makes for more efficient bowel movements. It also attracts water which helps keeps things softer and facilitates and easier passage. Be sure to drink plenty of water to help move things along.

Magnesium comes in many forms. Magnesium glycinate is my favorite when it comes to constipation relief or in helping those with cramping and restless legs. Magnesium glycinate is a chelated form, which makes it the most bioavailable form of magnesium and will correct deficiencies faster than any other type.

Magnesium oxide is a non-chelated type of magnesium, bound to an organic acid or a fatty acid. This is my second favorite form of magnesium. It contains 60 percent magnesium, and has stool-softening properties. Although magnesium citrate can be effective as well, my first choices would be glycinate or oxide.

If you have never considered magnesium supplementation, try this first. Once you correct a magnesium deficiency, you may not need to go much further in eliminating your constipation issues.

Senna

Senna is a potent herb native to the Southeast and Central America. It is commonly used on a short-term basis to treat constipation. It comes in tablets, capsules and liquid forms. It is a common ingredient in many teas for dieting and constipation relief. I refer to these as poopy tea. It is also used to empty the bowels before surgery and certain medical procedures. Senna is in a class of medications called stimulant laxatives. It works by increasing activity of the intestines to cause a bowel movement.

Senna is extremely harsh as compared to other herbal remedies, but it is actually one of the very rare herbs that are FDA approved for constipation relief.

Although very effective in producing bowel movements, senna can be habit forming in individuals who have used this herb long-term. Many are unable to achieve regular bowel habits after habitual use. Another complication that is considered fairly harmless is Melanosis coli. Melanosis coli is the brown discoloration of the interior wall of the colon that occurs in individuals who frequently use senna. This condition can be seen during a routine colonoscopy.

Although very helpful at times, senna should be considered a backup plan and should not be used regularly.

Cascara Seragata

Cascara bark, native to the Pacific Northwest, has been used for centuries for its stimulant laxative effects. Like senna, this should only be used occasionally for constipation.

Pregnant women should not use cascara, as it may have labor stimulating qualities. Those with IBS, colitis, Crohn's, hemorrhoids or kidney problems would be wise to avoid cascara as well.

Cascara was a popular ingredient in many commercially prepared laxatives that was FDA approved up until May of 2002. Although no longer FDA approved, cascara is still widely available in the herbal community.

Thought to be less habit forming than some of its herbal competitors, cascara is still a popular ingredient in many bowel-cleansing formulas. Like senna, Melanosis-coli is a potential side effect of regular use.

Cascara has its place in treating constipation, but regular use should be avoided.

Chlorophyll

Chlorophyll is the green pigment that makes it possible for plants to convert carbon dioxide and water into oxygen and glucose with the help of some sunlight (photosynthesis).

Chlorophyll is an excellent resource for those who want to build better blood quality, as well as improve the inner working of the digestive system. Chlorophyll promotes formation of hemoglobin and red blood cells. This may be very beneficial to anyone who has been told they have anemia. Hemoglobin is the iron-containing substance that provides blood with its red color and is responsible for transporting oxygen to all areas of the body.

While it is quite obvious that green foods are rich

in chlorophyll, benefits deteriorate during the cooking process. This is why supplementation should be considered.

For the constipated individual, chlorophyll loosens and cleanses the colon. Even though it is not considered a constipation remedy by itself, I have witnessed dramatic improvement in individuals who choose to supplement with chlorophyll.

As mentioned in a previous chapter, chlorophyll treats bad breath by deodorizing the digestive tract from deep within. When the inside of the body is cleansed and deodorized, the exterior parts of the body are deodorized as well. Body odor and stinky feet can be a thing of the past.

Chlorophyll has other benefits to the body. These include mineral balance, detoxification, and anti-infective and anti-inflammatory properties.

Anyone would benefit from chlorophyll, and there are no safety concerns. For those who lack in green food consumption, you'd be wise to consider adding this to your supplement regime. Dosing varies, but I would recommend it be taken twice daily to clean things up. Oh, and don't be alarmed at the new green color of your poop, it's all good!

Rhubarb

What many people don't know is that rhubarb is actually a vegetable. But in 1947, a New York court decided it was to be considered a fruit because it was used as a fruit. So a fruit it is.

Rhubarb has celery-like stalks and is well known for its very tart taste. Many are unaware that rhubarb can be used as a strong laxative and actually has been for approximately 5000 years. You will find it on the ingredient list of many herbal preparations designed for colon cleansing.

Some may benefit from using it in a smoothie. You may use honey or fruit to sweeten up the tart taste. Do not use the leaves, as these are poisonous. Use two to three stalks, chopped; and then blend with a cup of apple juice.

Ginger

Ginger is frequently mentioned in regards to its diverse healing potential. It is most noted for its protection against motion sickness.

For those who suffer from the discomforts of constipation, the carmative benefits of ginger will provide some relief. Ginger is an excellent carmative. Carmatives help the body get rid of uncomfortable gas pains. Ginger contains properties that stimulate the digestive process by increasing the wavelike motion called peristalsis. Those suffering from frequent cramping will find relief, as ginger has antispasmodic properties that help to soothe intestinal discomfort.

Ginger comes in a variety of forms, including fresh, dried, capsuled, crystallized, candied, pickled and powdered; all easily found in your fresh food market. Raw is always best for treating intestinal woes as compared to capsules, which seem to work best for motion sickness.

Triphala

Probably one of my personal favorites, triphala, is

something that I personally take but would hesitate to promote for my lack of Ayurvedic education. I feel it is balancing, energizing and improves my overall vitality. I just didn't know enough about its origin to recommend it comfortably to my clientele.

A few years back, I had the pleasure of meeting an Ayurvedic physician in Arizona. We were discussing what I did for a living and the topic of supplementation came up. I had previously taken triphala and told her how much I loved it. She reminded me that it would be an excellent choice for my clientele as it provides the body with gentle detoxification and cleansing. After reassuring me that anyone can take it, I now felt comfortable in recommending it in my practice.

Triphala literally means "three fruits". This combination herb originated in India and is currently used as a complete body cleanser. Not only does triphala detoxify and cleanse the colon, it also purifies the blood and facilitates the removal of toxins form the liver. Thiphala is also considered a potent antioxidant, as it contains impressive amounts of vitamin C.

Triphala is gentle and does not cause the cramping and urgency like other cleansing agents. Dosage varies per individual, though it is generally safe for all.

Psyllium

Psyllium is a soluble fiber used primarily as a gentle bulk-forming laxative in products such as Metamucil. It comes from a shrub-like herb called Plantago ovata that grows worldwide, but is most common in India. You can think of psyllium as little brooms that sweep the lining of the colon, but the colon needs to be moving for this to work well.

Psyllium husks can help lower cholesterol. It can help relieve both constipation and diarrhea, and is used to treat irritable bowel syndrome, hemorrhoids, and other intestinal problems. Psyllium has also been used to help regulate blood sugar levels in people with diabetes. When psyllium husk comes in contact with water, it swells and forms a gelatinous mass that helps transport waste through the intestinal tract. Use caution, as this may cause an uncomfortable backlog (literally) in those who are already constipated. For this reason, it is very important to get things "moving" before incorporating psyllium. There are a few very effective fiber blend products that utilize psyllium along with other herbs to promote cleansing as well as laxative effects.

Dried Fruit

All dried fruits, including prunes, raisins, figs, apricots, and dates, are beneficial when it comes to preventing and relieving constipation. Like other foods for constipation, they contain a lot of fiber, but they also contain other compounds that are very effective as natural laxatives and have stimulant properties. All dried fruits contain very good amounts of magnesium, which in itself stimulates bowel movements.

Prunes, also known as dried plums, are probably the most popular died fruit when it comes to constipation. High in both soluble and insoluble fiber, prunes soak up water, making stools bulkier and easier to pass. Some individuals prefer to soak and rehydrate the fruit first. In the constipated individual, this may initially cause some intestinal drama and discomfort. However, the excellent results that are likely to follow make it well worth it.

Although prunes and other dried fruits provide food for the healthy bacteria in the large intestine, one must also be aware of the higher sugar content. For fiber content, the actual fruit is better than just drinking prune juice.

Flaxseed

Also known as linseed, flaxseed is very high in fiber and rich in beneficial omega-3 fatty acids; both of which are helpful for constipation.

Each tablespoon of flaxseed contains 1gram of fiber. It has a sweet, nutty taste and can be added to almost anything. It's great in salads, cereals, and I have even added it to meatballs and turkey burgers.

Whole flaxseed provides little omega-3 benefit because your digestive tract is unable to crack open the hard shells that surround the seeds (which is where all the benefits are). But for constipation, even the whole seed may provide benefit as it forms a mucolytic coating that has a slip-sliding effect though the intestinal tract. Be sure to drink plenty of water to wash it down. If you grind your flaxseed, do so in small amounts, as the omega-3 benefit will dissipate after time. Keep it refrigerated once it has been ground.

Flaxseed deserves a little time in the spotlight as it has other benefits we have not yet discussed. Flaxseed is an excellent source of omega-3 for vegetarians or vegans, who use it in place of fish oils.

If lowering your cholesterol is a goal, ground flaxseed has been shown to work just as well as statins. Flaxseed contains high levels of lignans, which may play a very protective role against cancer, especially estrogen-dominant cancers. It has helped to normalize estrogen levels in post-menopausal women, which has many physical benefits as well as emotional. Flaxseed is also a good source of magnesium.

Flaxseed is currently involved in numerous studies that are showing promises ranging from heart disease to cancer. It is inexpensive and very easy to incorporate into your diet. I recommend consuming two ground tablespoons daily.

Chia Seed

Chia seeds are becoming more popular and are now easily found in the health food section of most grocery stores. Chia seed is the common name for Salvia hispanica. It is a species of a flowering plant in the mint family, native to central and southern Mexico and Guatemala. Up until now, chia seeds were most known for the popular Christmas gift, the Chia Pet. The chia seed was spread and sprouted over a terra cotta figure, and would resemble hair in just a few weeks.

Constipated individuals should consider the use of chia seeds, as they absorb ten times their weight in water, which forms a bulky gel. This bulky gel will travel through your digestive system with greater ease, making it less likely to become a hard, unmoving blockage.

Those attempting to lose weight will benefit, as chia seed reduces cravings and may prevent some calorie absorption. Chia seed will make you feel full as well as provide some hydrating benefit.

Chia seeds are a great source of omega-3 fatty acids. They actually contain more omega-3 than salmon.

This provides the body with beneficial anti-inflammatory properties.

Because chia seeds slow down how fast our bodies convert carbohydrates into simple sugars, studies indicate that they can help control blood sugar. This leads scientists to believe chia seeds may have great benefits for diabetics.

Chia seeds are easier to digest than flaxseed, and don't need to be ground up.

For those suffering from chronic constipation, this recipe has helped many individuals. Mix 1/3 cup of chia seeds with 2 cups of pure water. Wait approximately 5 minutes and stir the mixture again, as it will have thickened a bit. Drink it down. Now go check a mirror, as you will have to get some of those black seeds out from between your teeth. Drinking a large glass of water after taking the chia seeds will help wash them down. Every day (or night if you wish) take 2 tablespoons. It actually does not taste bad at all, and I have had many clients love the texture of the seeds. Be patient. If your constipation is chronic or severe, it may take three to six days before you experience soft, painless and productive bowel movements.

For individuals suffering from inflammatory conditions such as gout or arthritis, mix one to two tablespoons of chia seed in two ounces of organic, unsweetened cherry juice. I always let the chia sit for a while before drinking it down.

Pumpkin Seeds

Pumpkin seeds have many nutritional benefits, but for the purpose of this book I'm going to discuss its anti-parasitic qualities. Parasites are a common complication of the constipated individual.

Contrary to popular belief, including my own, parasites are not actually killed by pumpkin seeds. In actuality, intestinal worms appear to be paralyzed by them, which then makes them unable to hold onto the intestinal wall or constipated stool.

You can eat pumpkin seeds in any amount you wish, but to get the best benefit you may want to try the following:

Put a 3/4-cup of raw pumpkin seeds in a blender and add rice or almond milk to make a smooth paste. You can add a touch of honey or molasses if you wish for taste, but it is actually not that bad. You may have trouble finishing this, as it is very filling; so try half and follow with the second half 30 minutes later.

Drink a 16-ounce glass of water within 30 minutes of finishing the pumpkin seed mixture. To help maximize benefits, take a weight appropriate dose of food grade castor as well. Castor oil is a potent stimulant laxative that is typically fast acting (more on this topic in the next section). It would be wise to keep your toilet open and available. For those not wanting to take castor oil, Cape Aloe capsules taken before the pumpkin seed mixture may help move the paralyzed parasites through in a timely manner.

It is important that you are not constipated when you eliminate your parasites with the use of this pumpkin seed remedy. Get things moving first, and then incorporate this effective remedy to rid yourself of these intestinal critters.

Calcium Bentonite Clay

Although I do not typically recommend Calcium Bentonite clay (Living Clay) specifically to treat constipation, it often becomes a very valuable tool when it comes to detoxification and improving digestive health.

Our bodies are bombarded with toxins coming at us from all directions: the air we breathe, the food we eat, the water we drink, the cleaning products we use, and the byproducts of our own cellular waste that builds up inside us. Add constipation to the list, and we could be compared to a toxic waste site.

For those who have never heard of Bentonite clay or its benefits, keep reading, as you will likely want this multitasker close at hand. Bentonite clay is medicinal powdered clay that comes from weathered volcanic ash. Bentonite clay is one of the most effective natural intestinal detoxifying agents available and has been used as a potent healing agent for centuries throughout the world.

This liquid clay (or reconstituted powder), once inside our digestive system, is able to absorb an impressive amount of toxins such as heavy metals, free radicals and pesticides. It can be compared to a sponge that sops up a sloppy mess, absorbing many times its molecular weight in toxic matter. It also pulls toxins through the skin when applied topically in clay baths or in poultices. I have personally witnessed burns that healed faster than usual with topical applications. Gum disease and bacterial infections of the mouth are easily treated with just a twice a day swish and swallow.

Toxins tend to be positively charged whereas Bentonite clay is negatively charged. The two come together like a magnet and are easily eliminated via a healthy bowel movement, which, by the way, comes with greater ease and frequency in those who consume the clay. Most healing (from any cause) is accelerated by detoxification of the body, and Bentonite clay is one of many avenues one can take. In as little as two weeks, ingesting small amounts of liquid clay daily can improve intestinal irregularity as well as provide relief from chronic constipation, diarrhea, indigestion and ulcers. Ran Knishinsky, author of *The Clay Cure*, reported that drinking clay helped him eliminate painful ganglion cysts (non-cancerous tumors attached to joints and tendons) within two months, without surgery. My personal experience was settling an upset stomach with just one dose, which is one of the most common uses.

It has also proven to be a very beneficial tool when it comes to resolving diarrhea, calming colitis, and diverticulitis relief. I have even seen it help those suffering from Crohn's disease:

> *If being diagnosed with Crohn's disease at the ripe age of 18 wasn't the biggest sign that I was constipated in my health, I don't know what was. I don't mean physically, because my fellow "Crohnie's" would generally agree that constipation is RARELY (if ever) an issue. But when you have no physical symptoms your entire life and then wake up one day with an autoimmune disease, I think it's inevitable to say your general health has become a bit constipated.*

Thankfully, there was only a 10-month gap between the time I was diagnosed with Crohn's disease and the day I stumbled upon Cathi Stack at Journey II Health. (Which in my opinion, was still 10 months too many!) Cathi taught me the importance of diet and supplementation, while others in the medical field were still insisting that diet played no part in Crohn's disease. Yeah...okay.

After a tough battle, (which is unfortunately still ongoing); frequent changeups of medications, including antibiotic, steroid, TNF blocker and immunosuppressant drugs; I've pretty much concluded that my body doesn't want to "mask" Crohn's. No medication ever seems to provide relief— aside from the dreaded prednisone, which is my arch nemesis!

Cathi has done extensive research in putting me on quality supplement regimens for Crohn's, which we're forced to switch up often when my body gets too used to one. She's the type of person you just trust; she knows her "shit." Literally.

Though I trust Cathi with my life, I will admit that I was very skeptical and turned off when she introduced me to Calcium Bentonite clay. I usually don't question any of her recommendations, but she wanted me to drink dirt? Literally...mud? No thank you! Looking back now, I'm glad she was insistent with me. Calcium Bentonite clay is now my absolute favorite product to have on hand, and I don't go far without it. If you can throw back a shot of alcohol, you can throw back a shot of clay.

Within the first two days of drinking it, I felt like I did before I woke up with this horrible disease. Actually, I felt better than that. Maybe it was from the detoxification that was taking place, or maybe it was the calming effect it had on my digestive tract. Whatever it was, I will not question it. My energy level was up the most it had been in two years, and I was going to the bathroom regularly. What more could a girl ask for?

They also say that the body heals from the inside out, and I experienced that firsthand. The bumps on my forehead and cheeks, which I assume were from medications and toxic buildup in my body, disappeared within days of ingesting the clay. I'm glad I was able to learn through my own experience at a young age that a clean environment on the inside reflects to the outside as well.

The total effect that Calcium Bentonite clay has on the body has made me a personal advocate for life. I'd say it's the best use of clay since Gumby!

Besides the benefits from the ailments listed above, most individuals will notice a surge in physical energy, a clearer complexion, improved gum health, whiter eyes, and a stronger immune system.

The best way to drink Bentonite clay is on an empty stomach or at least one hour before or after a meal. It has little to no taste and is very easy to take. For those on prescription medications, it is recommended that you wait 1-3 hours before ingesting the clay, as not to interfere with medication absorption.

One of the better and more informative websites that has many articles and studies, including references, can be found at www.aboutclay.com. Do some of your own investigating and decide for yourself. I have seen many individuals benefit from the use of Bentonite clay.

OILS

Oils used for constipation relief fall under a category of products called lubricants, or emollients. The oil coats the stool, allowing it to become more "slippery" and therefore easier to pass through the digestive system. Consistently incorporating two tablespoons of oil to your diet per day would be of benefit, especially if it is taken all at once.

Olive Oil

Olive oil is well known for its omega-3 benefits, but people may not give it much thought in regards to constipation relief. Maybe they should. Unlike mineral oil, there are no adverse side effects and can be taken safely on a daily basis. Because of the strong taste, some individuals may have a hard time ingesting enough to make a noticeable difference in poop performance.

Besides the anti-inflammatory and cardio protective effects, olive oil provides additional perks to gastrointestinal health.

Mineral Oil

Mineral oil can interfere with the absorption of certain vitamins and minerals because it coats the intestines. It is best not to be taken regularly. I will admit to recommending it from time to time for the stubborn case of constipation, but never on a regular basis.

Commercial preparations are readily available. Typical doses are one to three tablespoons, and results are usually noticed within six to eight hours. Many choose to take this at bedtime.

Flaxseed Oil

Flaxseed oil has many of the same benefits as olive oil, and you may prefer this taste. The downside is that flax is not stable at room temperature and can become rancid; therefore flaxseed oil needs to be refrigerated. If you choose to take it for constipation, take one to three tablespoons before breakfast.

Castor Oil

Castor Oil is most well known for its ability to act as a stimulant laxative to ease constipation. The components in castor oil act to stimulate the walls of both the small and large intestines, which sets it apart from other oils. It creates purgative action in the colon, which works to move impacted fecal matter through in order to relieve symptoms associated with constipation.

It only takes a few hours to feel the benefits of castor oil. This is not always the most comfortable situation, as cramping and diarrhea are common. Dosage varies and it is very important that you follow directions on the bottle. Dosing recommendation range from one teaspoon to two tablespoons as an adult dosage. Castor oil can be mixed with a small amount of juice to improve the taste.

Castor oil should not be used in individuals who have an intestinal blockage, appendicitis, or other acutely painful situations. The effects of castor oil can be a bit more harsh than other oils when taken internally, and should not be taken for more than five consecutive days.

Castor oil applications vary. One of my midwifery instructors used to recommend it in early labor to speed things up in first time moms. The one and only time I had recommended this to a first time mom in early labor, I missed the delivery. She told me later that she had experienced intense diarrhea and cramping during labor. Labor is hard enough; I'm not sure if I'd like to add diarrhea and intestinal cramping to the mix. There are websites and blogs that recommend castor oil for the induction of labor. This will not work. The mom needs to be in early labor for this to work. I personally think it makes for a very intense labor.

Castor oil as a topical remedy is also popular, which will be discussed in the next chapter.

SUMMARY

Constipation is something the medical community does not give too much attention. Sadly, many are told that having bowel movements every two to three days is normal. Many well-intending physicians admit that they just don't know what else to do. Thank goodness the long-term solution is now within your reach, and doesn't require the help of your physician. It just takes time and patience.

Because of the way constipation makes you feel, it's probably difficult to imagine being able to work up the energy to focus on solving your own problem. If you want real, long-term relief, and wish to live a life full of energy and vitality, free of constipation and the woes that come with it, it's up to you to tweak your lifestyle in order to achieve success.

Use the information given above. Don't do everything, but start with something that you intuitively gravitate to. Then start filling your toolbox. The chronically constipated individual will need to switch things up from time to time.

Take charge of your own health and implement what has been effectively relieving constipation for thousands of years. Better yet, change your lifestyle to reflect a time long before constipation even existed.

Chapter 6

Therapies That "Move" You

COLON HYDROTHERAPY

I had no intention of adding colon hydrotherapy to my list of services when I began to pursue my career as a naturopath. But as I have stated previously, I cannot imagine helping people without it.

Many critics, including one of my favorite mentors from a distance, Dr. Oz, are not proponents of colon hydrotherapy. The general opinion is that it is unnatural to put water into the colon. I might agree, if what people were putting into their mouths were natural. Compared to purified water in the colon, what many people put in their mouths horrifies me.

Colon hydrotherapy is a safe, effective method for cleansing the colon of waste material by repeated, gentle flushing with filtered water at a comfortable temperature. It is also a means of hydration, as one of the main functions of the colon is to absorb water. I personally cannot imagine life without them.

The use of colon hydrotherapy in the treatment of

disease can be dated back to 1500 B.C. where it was first recorded in ancient Egyptian writings, the Ebers Papyrus. These types of enemas were described in those times as water infusions into the large intestine through the anus. Hippocrates recorded the use of enemas as a successful therapy for fever relief.

Despite considerable research in the early part of the century documenting its therapeutic effectiveness, it continues to be a highly controversial and often misunderstood form of therapy. In all my research, interest and experience in natural health, I have come to know the following; if the colon is not eliminating properly, all of the supplements, medications and therapies in the world will not be effective to their fullest potential.

A balanced state of wellness cannot be achieved in a constipated individual. What's normal? —Two to three bowel movements daily. Many individuals would consider this diarrhea or assume they must be sick. Let me ask you this. If you eat three to four meals daily and only go once per day, and have a hard time at that, where is it going? The average individual carries eight to fifteen pounds of solid fecal matter (poop) at any given time— ouch!

Discomfort, pain, bloating and gas are symptoms that so many experience when they are not "moving" normally. This backed-up material is quite toxic. Long-term buildup of material in the colon wall can inhibit muscular action causing sluggish bowel movements, an over-distended colon, and chronic constipation. The longer this is left unattended the harder it is to return to normal function—but it is possible; I see it all the time.

Bowel toxicity is prevalent in all civilized

societies, particularly in North America. The Standard American Diet (SAD) consists mainly of processed, manufactured and chemical laden foods. Signs of bowel toxicity include headaches, backaches, constipation, fatigue, bad breath, body odor, dark circles under the eyes, irritability, confusion, acne, abdominal gas and bloating, diarrhea, sciatic pain and so forth. Know anyone?

Herbal laxatives, enemas and suppositories may be helpful as quick fixes, but do little in the long-term to return the colon back to normal function. Dependency on these items is often created. Colon hydrotherapy actually helps restore normal peristalsis and colon function. The amount of visits does vary depending on the severity and duration of issues.

Although initially awkward, receiving a colonic is not painful or embarrassing. A qualified colon therapist will easily guide you through this experience. There is no odor or mess. If you explore more progressive areas of the country you will find that colon hydrotherapy is commonplace, especially for professional athletes and those who need to maintain a higher level of functioning and wellness.

Dorothy is a 68 year-old woman who shares her story about colon hydrotherapy:

> *I will begin as to why I started coming to Journey II Health. I was probably constipated for years and never realized or thought about it. Then about two years ago, I noticed large balls floating in the toilet after my bowel movements and then knew that was not normal. A good friend of mine*

told me about Journey II Health and colon cleansing and how Cathi helped a friend of hers. She said Cathi found parasites and helped her to get rid of them.

I remember my first visit and our talk. I came initially for five weekly treatments in the beginning and saw how constipated I was, and that my colon was enlarged and "plugged," if that is the right word. Cathi found parasites and I even saw them. She gave me medication to help get rid of them. I also started to take Cape Aloe on a daily basis. I continued my colon cleansing every five weeks.

It has been two years now and I feel so much better. I do get constipated from time to time, but I can now correct that problem so it does not get as bad as I was. I've lost some weight from all the waste that was in my colon. I've also learned from Cathi how important it is to take probiotics and Vitamin-D daily.
I've learned from Cathi the foods that can cause constipation and try to avoid them. My goal is to get my colon back to its normal size.

I find drinking warm water with a fresh squeezed lemon upon wakening in the morning helps to move your bowels.

In closing I want to say, "Thank you, Cathi, for helping me with my constipation and in feeling much better." The one hour I spend with Cathi every five weeks is priceless to me and flushing warm water in the colon and watching the waste leave my body makes me feel better, knowing it isn't remaining stagnant in my colon. I hope anyone reading this that has serious constipation problems will consider colonics. Colon cleansing is painless and all natural. It has changed my lifestyle.

Here is the information we give to our clients in order to explain what to expect during a typical colon hydrotherapy session…

Properly applied colon therapy consists of more than simply flushing the bowel. It involves a thorough, individual assessment including evaluation of environmental, immunological and psychosomatic influences. Based on this information, the appropriate therapeutic procedures are discussed and executed. The goals of colon therapy are as follows:

- To bring about efficient elimination of waste
- To restore tissue and organ function
- To rebalance overall body chemistry
- To teach clients to be responsible for their own health

141

Common Questions and Answers

- *What is colonic irrigation?*

Also known as a "colonic", "colon lavage", "colon
hydrotherapy", or "high colonic", colon irrigation is a
safe, effective method for cleansing the colon of waste
material by repeated, gentle flushing with filtered water
that is a comfortable temperature. In a 30 to 45 minute
session, as much as 20 to 35 gallons of water is used to
gently flush the colon. Through appropriate use of
massage, pressure points, reflexology, breathing
techniques, suggestion, etc., the colon therapist is able to
loosen and eliminate far more toxic waste than any other
short-term technique. Having an experienced colon
therapist available can be compared to having a
professional mechanic repair your automobile's engine.
The second and subsequent colonics will remove more.
How many and how often will depend on your personal
objectives. We have found that the majority of chronically
constipated individuals need approximately six colonics,
with no longer than one week between visits. The same
results may be achieved if you did 3-4 colonics over 1-1.5
weeks.

- *What is the colon and what does it do?*

The colon, also known as the large intestine, is the end
portion of the human digestive tract. The colon is
approximately five feet long and two inches in diameter.
Most of us have distended our colons to a larger
dimension, and therefore act as holding tanks for a large
amount of fecal matter. The main functions are to

eliminate waste and conserve water.

• *What is the purpose of having a colonic?*

Waste material, especially that which has remained in the colon for some time (i.e. impacted feces, dead cellular tissue, accumulated mucus, parasites, worms, etc.) will predispose you to many problems. First, this material is quite toxic (poisonous). These poisons can reenter and circulate the bloodstream making us feel ill, tired or weak. Second, impacted materials impair the colon's ability to assimilate minerals and bacteria-produced vitamins. And finally, build-up of material on the colon wall can inhibit muscular action causing sluggish bowel movements, constipation and the results of these disorders.

• *How can I tell if I have toxic material in my colon?*

Common signs include headaches, backaches, constipation, fatigue, bad breath, body odor, irritability, confusion, acne, abdominal gas and bloating, diarrhea, sciatic pain and more. As you can see, intestinal toxicity is part and parcel of many people's everyday experience.

• *Why not use enemas, suppositories or laxatives instead?*

Well, everything has its proper place, but most of those things really aren't substitutes for colonics. Enemas are useful for emptying the rectum, the lowest 8-12 inches of the colon. Usually, one or two quarts of water are used to do that. Suppositories are intended to accomplish the same task. Laxatives, particularly herbal laxatives, are formulated for constipation and/or to build up the tone of the colon muscle. The Rolls Royce of colon cleansing, without question, is colonic irrigation.

- *What will colonics do to the colon?*

1. Cleanse the colon. Toxic material is broken down so it can no longer harm your body. Even fecal material that has been built up over time is gently and surely removed in the process during a series of irrigations. Once impacted material is removed, your colon will begin to cooperate as it was meant to. In this very real sense, a colonic is a rejuvenation treatment.

2. Exercise the colon muscles. The build-up of toxic debris weakens the colon and impairs its functioning. The gentle filling and emptying of the colon improves peristaltic (muscular contractility) activity by which the colon naturally moves material.

3. Reshape the colon. When problem conditions exist in the colon, they tend to alter its shape, which in turn causes more problems. The gentle action of the water, coupled with the massage techniques of the colon therapist, helps to empty bulging pockets within the bowel and helps to widen narrowed, spastic constrictions. This enables the colon to resume to its natural state.

4. Stimulate reflex points. Every system or organ in the body is connected to the colon reflex points. Colonic

irrigation stimulates these points, thereby affecting the corresponding body parts in a beneficial way (similar to reflexology).

- *What are the additional benefits I might expect from a colonic?*

There are many benefits you can expect. You will learn to expand your awareness of your body's functioning by listening to signals from your abdomen, skin, face, and even your bowel habits. You will spot conditions early before they become something more severe.

The solar plexus is the emotional center of the body and the transverse colon passes right through it. If an emotional event is left uncompleted, it often results in physical tension being stored in the solar plexus, which affects all organs in this area, including the colon. This results in constipation. Not only do colonics relieve constipation, they can assist you in recognizing and releasing the stored emotions causing the problem.

Other benefits of colon hydrotherapy include decreased gas and bloating, increased alertness, more frequent bowel movements, decreased mucus, detection of parasites, and clarification of the whites of the eyes. It clears the skin; minimizes age and liver spots; helps to minimize withdrawal from drugs, alcohol and nicotine; improves mood; lessens symptoms associated with PMS, menopause and depression; minimizes allergies; decreases the occurrence of headaches; and reduces and even eliminates symptoms associated with IBS (Irritable Bowel Syndrome), diverticulosis and a spastic colon.

- *Is a colonic painful?*

It rarely is. Usually, painful experiences are the result of resistance and tension. A professional colon therapist is skilled at putting you at ease and minimizing any discomfort. Most people enjoy the colonic and are especially pleased with the sensation of feeling lighter, clean and clearer afterward. Sometimes during a colonic, the colon muscles will contract and suddenly expel considerable amounts of liquid and waste into the rectum. This may be precipitated by a brief episode of cramping and/or urgency. Such episodes, if they occur, are brief and easily tolerated.

- *Is it embarrassing to get a colonic?*

NO! You will fully maintain your personal dignity. You will be in a private room with only your therapist, who fully appreciates the sensitivity of this procedure and will help you feel at ease. Your emotions are acknowledged, as we realize this may be initially awkward. After the gentle insertion of the small tube into the rectum, you are completely covered. Single-use tubing in a closed system brings clean water in and carries waste out. There is no odor and no mess with a colonic.

- *How do I prepare for a colonic?*

Water consumption and a clean diet will help pave the way. Real foods such as fruits, vegetables, nuts and seeds help produce the best results. If your diet is less than perfect, we recommend a light diet of fruits, vegetables and whole grains the day before. On the day of your colonic, avoid eating two hours prior to your procedure—but drinking water and herbal teas are OK. If your colonic is very early, it is OK to eat lightly. Remember: There is an abdominal massage involved. You wouldn't want that on a full stomach.

* *What can I expect afterwards?*

Most likely you will feel great. You will probably feel lighter and enjoy a greater sense of well being. Someone getting his or her first colonic usually remarks that it was one of the most wonderful experiences of their life. Any activity you would ordinarily do, such as work or exercise, is fine to do afterwards. For some, the colonic may trigger several subsequent bowel movements for the next few hours, but there won't be any uncontrollable urgency or discomfort. It's also possible to feel chilled for a few minutes after a colonic. Many people come during their lunch break and I am willing to bet that they are more productive for the second half of their day.

* *Why would a series of colonics be beneficial?*

It is important that you be aware of your objective when working with a colon therapist. For example, if your objective is to recover from the flu, lower a fever, or relieve lower back pain; one or two colonics may be all you need. However, perhaps your objective is to overcome a life-long habit of constipation, to learn to create multiple daily bowel movements, or to achieve vital health; to do this may require regular colonics, as well as dietary, exercise, and attitudinal changes. How many depends on the condition of your body and how well it responds to treatment. One size doesn't fit all as far as treatment recommendations.

- *Are colonics dangerous?*

Being an essentially natural process, there is virtually no danger with a colonic. The intent is to provide a safe and health promoting service. Our products are sterile and we adhere to strict guidelines in the upkeep of our equipment. Purified water free of chlorine and sediment is mandatory. Chlorine destroys good bacteria in the colon.

- *Will colonics upset the electrolyte balance?*

The majority of material released during a colonic is formed stool has that already had the fluids and electrolytes removed from it. So the amount lost is very minimal and easily replaced by the body from the food and fluid we ingest.

- *Will colonics wash out my beneficial intestinal flora (healthy bacteria) and nutrients?*

The truth is that washing out putrefied material from the large intestine, which is only partially reached in any colon irrigation, INCREASES the good intestinal flora. Good bacteria can only breed in a clean environment. We highly recommend you take probiotics while investing the time and money in cleaning out your colon. Our facility provides a dose following each treatment—

but we also recommend daily use.

• *Will having colonics help improve my immune system?*

The removal of old stagnant waste and toxic residue could rejuvenate the immune tissue that resides in the intestines. Recent European studies speculate that 80 percent of the immune tissue resides in the intestines. This leads us to believe that this type of therapy could influence such immune deficiency diseases as cancer and AIDS. Colon hydrotherapy is not a cure-all, but an important adjunctive therapy in the overall health care of the client.

• *How long does a colonic take?*

Your first appointment will probably last 1.5 hours. The actual colonic procedure takes 35-45 minutes. There will be approximately 15 minutes prior to the session in which you will change and have a deep intestinal massage to maximize results. Results will be discussed during and after the procedure. Subsequent appointments should last about one hour.

• *Can I eat after having a colonic?*

We recommend that you eat a moderate amount of whatever seems gentle and nourishing to you. Just as it does not make sense to wash your car then drive through mud, eating a meal known to cause trouble is not an intelligent choice. Salads, vegetables, fruits, soups and broths are your best choices.

* *Will one colonic empty the colon?*

Almost never. First of all, many of us have impacted feces (hardened, rubbery or wall-like matter that weighs about 8-15lbs) in our colons. Substantial work must be done to remove it. One colonic will remove some of the stagnant waste. The second and subsequent colonics will remove more. Often, It takes as many as four to six colon hydrotherapy sessions to see and feel very dramatic results. Please note, your colon therapist is not dragging you through a series of unnecessary appointments. The state of your insides will determine the amount of sessions you will need, and most of us need at least four.

Procedure for First Colonic Irrigation

You will be asked about your medical history. Your goals, objectives and concerns will be discussed. You will be asked to undress from the waist down and will be given a gown or towel to cover up. You will need to empty your bladder. An abdominal massage will take place. Instructions will be given on how to lie on the table while gentle insertion of a rectal tube is accomplished. The filling and flushing of the colon begins. The waste material can be viewed by the client through a specially designed view tube (and believe me you will become fascinated). Cleansing lasts 35-45 minutes. The rectal tube is gently removed and you are given ample opportunity for a final visit to the bathroom.

Personal Experience

Many individuals and traditional healthcare professionals wonder if this is a safe procedure. I have worked in traditional medicine (and still do) for over 25 years and have never seen such dramatic improvement in overall health. If all hospitals and nursing homes provided this service, healing would be expedited and patients would require fewer pain medications. The elderly would not be as confused, as they would be able to metabolize their medications better. Clear thinking is a benefit of a clean colon! Pain medications often cause constipation, and therefore tend to complicate matters. IBS (Irritable Bowel Syndrome) is easily treated. I can assure you, many referrals come from physicians and surgeons that I personally work with. Strict health and safety guidelines are adhered to, so there is virtually no danger in the procedure.

As you probably have guessed, I am an advocate for colon hydrotherapy. I have personally been receiving treatments and providing this service for a number of years. Here is a very animated client, now friend, who describes her experience with colonics. Charmagne is a character (an actress as well) and I love her bluntness!

> *I LOVE COLONICS! I will tell anyone who will listen that they need to go see Cathi and have a colonic. And then go back and see her and have another one. Rinse and repeat forever.* (There are many highly qualified individuals across the country and even

worldwide who will help you—but thanks
Charmagne.)

*I struggled with constipation and GI issues
for YEARS. I would bounce between
extreme constipation followed by bouts of
diarrhea. Not fun. I just wanted to poop
once (or twice!) a day like a NORMAL
PERSON! I didn't think that was too much
to ask and Cathi didn't either.*

*My first colonic was exciting. Cathi
lubricated the tube and put it gently in my
ass and we were OFF! We found out I had
parasites as we watched my poop (and
parasites) fly by in the observation window
of the colon-hydrotherapy machine. And
don't judge me for being excited to see my
poop fly by. You will TOTALLY want your
colon hydrotherapist to get out of the way so
you can watch your poop fly by, too. It's
okay to admit you want to see it. We're all
friends here.*

*My offering to the colonic gods used to be
all hard and slow (and brown). After some
dietary tweaks (and regular colonics), I now
provide them with the brown-green soft stuff
they LOVE! In return for my offering, the
colon hydrotherapy gods recharge my
batteries for a few days. That's literally
what it feels like. The colonic exhausts me
in the short-term and then for days*

afterwards I feel like someone gave me a new battery.

I am happy to report that I now poop once or twice a day, except under conditions of extreme stress. THANKS, CATHI!

ENEMAS

Most people are familiar with enemas and have even had one sometime over the course of their lifetime. Used to clean the lower colon and rectum, this therapy is mainly used to treat constipation or detoxify the body in order to improve health.

Cool water enemas (50 -65 degrees) have been used for centuries to reduce fever. This is very effective and yet something that is often not considered anymore. The cooler water temperatures are also effective for those suffering from inflammatory bowel conditions such as colitis.

Most enemas can be done in the privacy of your own home, while some are performed under the supervision of a medical professional.

Cleansing Enema

These kits can be found at any drug store. The bags can be filled with 1.5-2 quarts of tepid water. I would avoid using tap water, as chlorine and fluoride have no place in the colon.

The enema bag is placed approximately four feet above where the individual will be lying down. Some prefer lying on their left side while others prefer knee-chest position. The key to success is to instill the water slowly. If you let the water in too fast, cramping is likely to end the session before adequate water has been placed. A gentle massage of the abdomen may help improve results. The goal is to hold for ten minutes or until the urge to defecate becomes too strong.

Sodium Phosphate or Saline Enema

These enemas are sold in most pharmacies in prepackaged disposable bottles with pre-lubricated tips. Easy to insert, these may be beneficial for situational constipation. Although the enema is not uncomfortable to receive, some have difficulty holding it in long enough to see benefit.

Occasionally, a pregnant patient, not in labor, presents extremely constipated to the labor wing. She is not in labor but uncomfortable due to constipation. The physicians typically do not know what to do. The following has worked well on more than one occasion: Insert Dulcolax suppository as directed. In twenty minutes, gently instill a slightly warmed prepackaged (Fleet) enema. I usually run the enema under luke warm tap water. Test it on your inner wrist to make sure it is not too hot. Typically, the constipated individual will be up to go to the bathroom within 15-20 minutes from the time the enema was given. The average person leaves the bathroom relieved and smiling. Results are often impressive.

Oil Enema

Usually mineral oil or castor oil enemas are found to be

useful in individuals who need to avoid straining or those unable to strain. The fecal matter will pass with greater ease and manual removal of stool is easier for those in a coma or incapacitated. Mineral oil enemas should be avoided on a regular basis, as they deplete nutrients by pulling out oil-soluble vitamins and minerals, which are then excreted into the feces.

Yogurt Enema

Yogurt enemas are sometimes recommended for treating irritable bowel syndrome, intestinal parasites and mild constipation. Plain yogurt contains live bacteria that regulate the digestive system and other parts of the body in cases of disease such as cancer and conditions including hemorrhoids. The Reflorestation enema (described below) is a much more effective version of the yogurt enema and far less messy.

Reflorestation Enema

Developed by colon guru Victoria Bowmann, PhD, the Reflorestation enema is a highly effective prepackaged kit that is easily instilled following reconstitution with water. It repopulates the colon with 50-billion multiple strains of healthy bacteria. This treatment is most effective on an empty colon so the best time would be following a colon hydrotherapy session or a series of sessions. The living bacteria are reconstituted with a small amount of water and inserted prior to bedtime. I have had many success stories from those that have included this therapy, especially in those suffering from IBS or chronic yeast conditions.

Barium Enema

Barium enemas are used to improve the visibility of the colon on X-rays during medical examinations. Single-contrast barium enemas utilize barium, while double-contrast barium enemas involve administering barium, draining most of the barium, and filling the colon with air to see narrowed regions, diverticuliti and other areas of inflammation in the colon.

Soapsuds Enema

Soapsuds enemas prove to be more effective at emptying the bowels for some people than water alone. If you want to experiment with your enema effectiveness, or don't find that your bowel empties well, add soap to your water. Always use a therapeutic, plant-based, animal-based, or food-based soap such as castile soap, chamomile and sage goat milk soap, or frankincense and myrrh goat milk soap.
    Please avoid the popular antibacterial soaps, or ones with chemicals such as sodium laureth sulfate, which is potentially carcinogenic (cancer causing). They are far too harsh for the delicate insides of the colon.

Coffee Enema

Coffee enemas are popular when it comes to detoxifying the body. This type of enema is worthy of your research efforts, and if you are ill you may want to investigate this further.
    The coffee enema was first rigorously used as a healing treatment by Dr. Max Gerson, MD, in the 1940s

and 1950s, to treat his cancer patients and is now the subject of serious scientific study in its promise and benefit for cancer patients.

Coffee enemas are used to increase the liver's detoxification capacity. Certain substances in the coffee stimulate an important detoxification enzyme in the liver, as well as dilate the bile ducts, increasing the flow of bile.

The pure filtered water, organic coffee, and unbleached coffee filter are essential for making a clean and safe solution. There are many resources available for more information on this topic, but I highly recommend gerson.org.

Enema Implants

Enema implants are therapeutic substances that may be used during or after a colon cleanse. Common enema implants could be chlorophyll, probiotics, Aloe Vera, coffee or any other substance that would benefit the individual by nourishing the tissue of the colon. They are often tolerated well and can be extremely therapeutic in a short period of time. They are easy to hold. Enema implants were the original way to hydrate the body before intravenous therapy became commonplace.

SUPPOSITIORIES

Suppositories are generally soft, bullet shaped supplements that are gently inserted into the rectum, where they melt and absorb easily into the colon wall. The most popular type of suppositories are listed below. Medications can also be in suppository form and are useful in those who cannot swallow, are vomiting, or are too young.

Glycerin Suppositories

Glycerin suppositories are one of the most widely used rectal laxatives for relieving mild to moderate constipation in babies, adults and children. Glycerin suppositories provide gentle, timely and effective relief from constipation with minimal side effects.

Dulcolax Suppositories

Dulcolax suppositories work by triggering the rhythmic muscles in your colon, helping to eliminate stool. Dulcolax suppositories are often preferred over oral laxatives because they don't pose the risk of interfering with nutrient absorption. Dulcolax suppositories also don't have the same uncomfortable side effects like nausea, gas and bloating or increased thirst. With a suppository, you will generally get a much more predictable and speedy result within 15-60 minutes. Dulcolax suppositories are also safe to use once a day, for seven days. The suppositories also dissolve organically, so there is no need to remove them once they have been inserted.

CASTOR OIL PACK

Many of the older and wiser elders are likely to be somewhat familiar with castor oil, but the memories of their mothers forcing it down their throats may not be pleasant. Fortunately, the benefits of castor oil are plentiful and you don't even have to swallow it.

There is an entire book on the benefits and almost miraculous applications of castor oil. Written by William A. McGarey, MD, "The Oil That Heals" reveals a large variety of successful castor oil treatments. From preventing abdominal surgery, to dissolving gallstones and even eliminating warts, this inexpensive lubricant has had some magical results. Might it have something to do with the origin of the oil? Castor oil comes from the Palma Christi plant, (the palm of Christ).

Application to puncture wounds several times per day, after washing, seems to potentiate healing and minimize scar formation. There have been many accounts of no scarring at all. It has also been reported that soaking in Epsom salts for 15 minutes each night, before applying the castor oil cloth, can eliminate toenail fungus. In as little as two months, the toenail returned back to normal. Anyone who suffers from this ailment knows that this is a very short period of time to resolve such a difficult issue.

One of the most popular applications is the infamous castor oil pack. Especially helpful in issues involving the gall bladder, liver, lymphatic and intestines, a castor oil pack involves the use of cloth soaked in castor oil, which is placed on the skin. Some alternative practitioners use it to enhance circulation and promote the healing of the tissues and organs underneath the skin.

To make a castor oil pack, soak a triple layer of un-dyed wool or flannel (12x18) in castor oil and simply place it on the skin. The flannel should be soaked, but not dripping. The flannel is covered with a sheet of plastic, and then a hot water bottle or heating pad is placed over the plastic to heat the pack. Leave on for approximately 60-90 minutes. The most common application is over the abdomen, especially concentrating on the right side (liver area). It can also be placed over inflamed and swollen joints. Be sure to rinse the area with a warm baking soda and water mixture when you are done to remove the residue from your skin. The soaked cloths can be kept in a plastic bag in the refrigerator and reused multiple times. You can reheat by placing in a low oven or placing it on the heating pad prior to application. Always check your temperature to avoid burns.

I have seen this application help with constipation, diarrhea, pancreatitis, menstrual cramping and abdominal discomfort in general. Although I can't explain how it works, I am constantly amazed at the results. In cases of severe abdominal pain, please see your doctor.

MASSAGE

Abdominal massage can absolutely improve bowel habits. Massage helps improve blood flow, tone and peristalsis (remember that inchworm-like motion?) within the colon.

Anyone can do it, and it can even be done to small infants. At our facility, we perform a gentle abdominal massage before and during each colon hydrotherapy session to facilitate the release of fecal matter—and it works. If you'd like to give it a try, the best time is before you get up in the morning (well maybe you should empty your bladder first) or even in the shower. You may use oil if you wish, but it is not necessary.

Start in the lower right corner of the belly and make small circular motions. This is the area of the ileocecal valve, the place where the small and large intestine come together. It is a one-way valve that often becomes dysfunctional in those suffering with constipation or intestinal parasites. Work your way up to almost the ribcage, across the upper abdomen (above the bellybutton) and then down the left side until you reach low into the left side. Most constipated individuals will feel more pressure on this side, as they have distended things a bit.

You will increase your chances of a successful, productive bowel movement if you make this a regular practice.

Chapter 7

CONSTIPATED Thoughts on Health

You Are Not Sick for Lack of a Pill

As a nurse midwife I have the opportunity to do many history and physicals, and there are definite patterns that have me screaming, "this is so obvious" in the back of my head. Chronic sinus conditions are related to food allergies more than 90 percent of the time. Dairy and gluten are very common denominators, and if the person has a blood type of "O" or "A", this is most likely the case. Blood typing is a standard test during pregnancy. So as they rattle off their history, so much of what ails them makes sense to me. Then there is acne and sensitivity to smells; chronic congestion leading them to their first allergy pill, until eventually it doesn't work anymore (because you haven't fixed the problem); and the chain of medications begins to grow.

How sad to find yourself at 50 or 60 years of age

and on three to five prescriptions. You are slowly being buried under side effects and medications that are curing nothing. They are pacifying what is not being fixed. Unfortunately, it is the rare patient that is given the nutritional advice that could actually reverse many illnesses.

Yes, there is a population of people who would rather have the doctor platter them up a pill rather than take any responsibility themselves, except of course to swallow that pill. YOU, not your doctor, must be the first one to take control and total responsibility for your own health. If you expect your doctor to take care of and fix everything, you are setting yourself up for disappointment.

A Good Doctor

There is no place I would rather be when it comes to great surgeons and excellent acute care medicine. I am sure I am not the only one that has witnessed near death traumas miraculously put back together to enjoy a life that could have easily been cut short. The surgical technology of today is beyond what most of our minds can conceive.

As frustrating as it may seem at times, you must try to remember that your doctor does want to help you. In a very limited amount of time, he or she will most likely be able to match a drug to the symptoms you are complaining of. If not, there will be blood work and possibly other diagnostic tests, the detective work begins, and hopefully an answer will be found. Unfortunately, most of my patients are frustrated when it comes to their medical care. They typically have 5-10 minutes to let their doctor know how they feel and reluctantly take the prescription that will hopefully cure what ails them. If you haven't already noticed, drugs typically don't cure you but do provide a nice Band-Aid. Over time, those drugs tend to create symptoms all of their own. Where we fail is finding the core of the problem, which usually has to do with the diet. We look at one organ system, and fail to view the body as a whole. All too frequently, we become lost in a pile of specialists.

Rarely will your health care provider have time to discuss your eating habits, bowel habits, and stress in your life and how they relate to what the problem is. This is where the system fails—big time. Don't blame your doctors; it was not part of their program. Digestive issues, wound healing, obesity, heart disease, skin conditions, adult onset diabetes, fungal infections, chronic sinusitis and cancer (just to name a few conditions) are all directly related to what goes into that mouth of yours.

If you really want to get well, live long, or experience a higher state of health, YOU need to facilitate it. The individual who expects to find it in his or her doctor's office will be very disappointed at no fault of the physician. Doctors are an easy target for blame when all goes awry. It doesn't matter that you left the office, lit a cigarette, and drove though the nearest fast-food chain; for some will still blame the health care provider for why they are not getting better.

There is an old Chinese Proverb that goes like this, "The superior doctor prevents sickness; the mediocre doctor attends to impending sickness; the inferior doctor treats actual sickness." A good doctor should not have an office full of sick people. If he or she is doing a great job, his or her patients should be infrequent visitors to the office.

Nutrition is the biggest failure when it comes to training our health care providers. I know this from personal experience. If it were common knowledge that sugar causes inflammation and prevents healing by feeding fungal conditions; artificial sweeteners are neurotoxic; and most individuals are allergic to dairy and sensitive to gluten—we'd be sick less and heal much faster. We need healthy fats to metabolize fat and provide the body with energy and organ protection. Most of us do not get enough healthy fats (omega-3's) in our diet.

I know for a fact it takes longer than a 10-minute appointment to customize an individual's eating plan. Contrarily, it only takes a minute or two to write a prescription that will likely provide relief in the short term, but overall did not fix the underlying problem.

When one takes on the entire responsibility for his or her health, they are likely to see dramatic improvements. Your doctor will then become an essential tool to help keep a watch over things. Even better, you will need fewer visits and medications as you will feel so much better and will only need routine check-ups. Routine lab work will serve only as a tool to keep you in check or to flag areas that need improvement.

You are your own best doctor when it comes to preventative medicine. Your well-intending doctor comes in very handy from time to time, but is not your best choice when it comes to preventing illness or nutritional guidance. Fortunately, there is a wealth of information available like never before and it is all within your reach. You need to read, research, or find the right person to guide you; for you my friend, are a worthy cause.

CONSTIPATED Health Care

What many individuals fail to realize as they call their doctors for every ache and pain, or show up at the local emergency room for a non-life-threatening event, is the unfavorable statistics within our own health care system.

Did you know that at least 187,000 people die each year in hospitals due to medical errors? 6.1 million suffer medical injury in and out of hospitals. 106,000 people die from medication taken as prescribed. These are scary numbers and I would hope you would do anything in your power to stay out of the hospital.

The irony of this all, is that I still work in a hospital. Yes, my co-workers and I do our best to create the best experience possible for our patients and are strong advocates when it comes to their care and safety. Fortunately, I work on a unit where the patients are pregnant, healthy and are on few medications. Most are discharged in a few short days.

Hospitals Fail When It Comes to Foods That Heal

I have been employed by various hospitals over the years, so what I am about to say is not directed toward any specific health care facility or person, it is a generalization and only meant to make you think.

If you are a patient in a hospital we can conclude a few possibilities. You are sick, having surgery, having a baby or mending from an accident. You have been placed in that facility to expedite the healing process, manage pain, and achieve a higher level of wellness—or at least that is what we are hoping for.

By now I hope most people have made the

connection between what you eat and your state of health. Your health, or lack of it, is largely determined by what you place in that mouth of yours. A diet full of raw fruits, vegetables, fish, beans, meats and whole grains is unlikely to yield you a candidate for diabetes, cancer or heart disease. A diet full of breads, cold cuts, macaroni and cheese, pizza, soda, chicken wings and subs are a fast-track to the diseases mentioned above, along with obesity and inflammatory issues.

So now you find yourself as a patient in a hospital. We are all likely to have this experience at some point in our life. Be it an accident, surgery or illness, we are all at risk.

Healing is expedited if the body is nutritionally supported. Pancakes, bagels, pudding and bread will absolutely slow the healing process as well as constipate you. Artificial sweeteners are as close to poison as you can get and should absolutely be banned from any institution that is promoting health. Carbonated beverages? How is phosphoric acid and carcinogenic (cancer causing) caramel coloring supposed to promote healing? So many people are suffering from digestive disorders but have no problem pouring this acid down their throat. These are just some of the foods that are responsible for destroying our health, and should be banned from any healing institution.

Slow wound healing is not the fault of the doctor, nurse, or any other health care professional. It has everything to do with the less than perfect state of the individual. A diet abundant with breads, processed and sugary foods is likely to be loaded with yeast. I can tell you from lots of experience, healing will not be accelerated. The risk for infection is dramatically increased when the body is lacking in healthy bacteria colonies and is loaded with yeast. It is easy to blame others when the healing is not going as planned, but it is truly the state of the individual that is to blame. Unfortunately, most dietitians have limited knowledge when it comes to foods that heal. But they are not to blame either. Food service companies are hired by the hospital and I am sure there are limited selections. Cost is a factor and poor food choices are cheaper than healthy choices. Processed foods have a shelf life, whereas fresh nourishing foods loaded with vitamins, minerals, and enzymes do not.

In my opinion, an institution that promotes healing would obviously not offer artificial sweeteners, MSG loaded soups and broths, and would keep the sugar to a bare minimum. Butter is the only option. Artificial, artery-clogging spreads, such as margarine, should never be offered. Hospitals would shorten patient stays if the focus would be nutrition based.

Wheatgrass shots, juicing, or healthy protein shakes (not ENSURE which is loaded with sugar) should be served to give energy and healing potential to those trying to heal. Juicing would maximize nutrition in a small volume that most patients would tolerate easily. Salad dressings should be olive oil and vinegar or lemon juice, and not a packet filled with chemicals. "Real" eggs should be served everyday in order to protect your "good cholesterol". American cheese, AKA plastic, has no place in any diet. Fake and artificially flavored yogurts should be avoided as well.

So what should you do? Be conscious to the food choices you make if you are trying to heal. Have family members or friends bring in healthy foods such as fresh salads and fruits. Homemade soups made from broths that do not contain MSG would provide the recovering individual with excellent nutrition that is easier to digest. Drink lots of pure filtered water.

No one wants an extended stay in the hospital. Studies show that the longer the stay, the higher the incidence of infection, complications, and even death. Nourish your body well and it will reward you with a speedy recovery.

As Thomas Edison once said...

"The doctor of the future will give no medicine, but will interest his patients in the care of the human frame, in proper diet, and in the cause and prevention of disease."

PART TWO

CONSTIPATION IN OTHER
AREAS OF YOUR LIFE

Y ou can choose to live in the world of your perceived past experiences and suffer there, OR you can choose to live in this world now—new, no judgment, no baggage. How liberating.

You Are Responsible For Most of the Emotional Clutter In Your Life

Our own belief systems usually prevent us from achieving our life aspirations, and then throw in the horrible state of our congested bowel—no wonder we feel like slugs by the time we reach our forties and fifties. The extra weight, the lack of energy, and the wonderful excuse of our hormones! Stop eating "crap" in the form of sugar and processed foods and watch those hormones balance. I dare you. Then let's add the ridiculously high numbers of people on antidepressants and this will "constipate" your life even more. Now I'm not insensitive to the occasional need for help during stressful life events, but I am opposed to long-term use. I am also VERY opposed to the use of antidepressants and antianxiety drugs without regular therapy. To me, the drugs will conveniently bury whatever it is that is causing your angst. Whereas a therapist, (a good one), will help bring issues to the surface rather than support your emotional constipation.

So many people sit unmoving in their life, waiting for happiness and fulfillment to just show up. This form of constipation involves the inability to make decisions or move forward in one's life. I know so many intelligent people who are stuck here. They lack the self-esteem and self-worth to move ahead. Sadly, no one else seems to understand why this person with so much potential can't seem to make a move. This is frustrating for all parties.

This next section pertains to the constipated areas of our social, emotional and spiritual lives.

Chapter 8

CONSTIPATED Relationships

In Love & War

A few years ago, one of my very closest friends told me to say at least one nice thing to my husband everyday. Now, if you ask him, he will say I have some catching up to do but I will say that this very simple tool has tremendous power. Compliments, praise and respect empower the receiver, and the giver will only get the same in return, tenfold.

When I began writing this book, I had a few close friends going through divorce. I watched as the pain etched away at them. It is so easy to get sucked into the pain of people you care about, and it is so easy to take sides. I will caution you here—that always backfires.

Somewhere between his and her side of the story lies the delicate truth. Each has interpreted the relationship differently and believes they have been wronged, or may actually be justifying their inappropriate behavior. The blame game begins, and there is rarely a winner.

If you and I were to interpret an event that we had witnessed together, we'd most likely have different perspectives. The gestures, body language, and tone would likely make our interpretations different.

Controlling Partners

The biggest downfall to any relationship is the controlling partner. Even if it is out of love, the controlled partner eventually feels trapped. If the situation is not remedied, that partner is likely to fly, or at least begin to feel crippled. This is my definition of a constipated relationship.

The scenario goes like this (and don't feel bad if this is you, there are millions out there who can relate): Low self-esteem Lucy meets controlling Ken. Ken actually loves Lucy but feels he has to keep everything in "order". As the provider, he sees himself in the dominant role. He does have the intention of wanting what's best. He wants a life with Lucy. He wants what is best for her and the children, and he takes the role as a "the provider" very seriously.

Lucy loves that she can depend on Ken. Ken makes her feel special. She does not mind keeping house, raising the kids, and letting Ken do as he wishes, because she is lucky to have someone who cares and supports her.

As the kids grow, she becomes less important and does not know who she is anymore. She knows this because Ken tells her from time to time that she would be nothing without him. These may not be the exact words, but it is the gist of things. Lucy begins to feel uncomfortable. With the kids becoming more independent, she wants to know who she is. Maybe she wants to work or start a business. She has been protected long enough, has raised her kids, and is now ready to spread her wings.

Ken is NOT ready for Lucy to do any such thing! He is the provider and has done a great job. Why would Lucy want anything else? How could she need anything else? THIS IS WHERE THINGS GET UGLY.

Ken was only doing his best, and Lucy seemed happy. What went wrong? Lucy will never deny that she was happy and grateful that Ken came into her life. The problem began when Lucy became ready to "step out" per say, and discover who she really is or what she was really meant to do. There is more to life than raising a family. I feel many of you cringing as you read this, and I know some are angry. But the truth is, 20 years goes by fast and that is not all there is to your life.

How do you let yourself fall into a rut so deep that your own hopes, dreams and potentials are tucked away, never to be your reality? Do you like who you are in your relationship? Does your relationship foster your own self-growth? How do you grow when you are unhappy and unfulfilled?

A great relationship is a two-way street. You give and you get. More importantly, you grow. A good relationship is not threatened by growth or a change in direction. A good partner enjoys watching the other grow. It may not always be easy, but the reward is priceless. Change is good. So many resist the change that will take you to a better place in your life. I'm not saying that your spouse has to change with you, rather accept and love you for who you are. We all grow at different rates, in different directions. Monogamy and loyalty to your current partner is essential in building a rock hard foundation. Nothing good comes from deceit, and nothing of substance and duration can be built on shaky ground.

You want to be WANTED, not NEEDED, and in order to be wanted, you have to be in a give-and-take relationship. What you give, you receive. This is true in everything but control. If you try to control, you get someone who will eventually spin out of control and most likely fly the coop. You give love—you get love. Love is not defined by anything material...ever.

Be wary of the person who says they love you and they only show it by keeping a roof over your head and providing for you. This is a dominant provider role, and even though it may be the only way they know how to love, it is not fulfilling.

People who love you make you feel good. They truly want to be with you but also give you the space you need to be who you are. Yes, they may feel threatened from time to time as you spread your wings, but they have nothing to worry about because if they weren't there to support your flight, you wouldn't be able to do it. This is the give and take of a good relationship.

Jealousy

Constipation in the form of jealousy is a form of insecurity that can and will be toxic to any relationship. Yes it may be cute at first, as you would interpret it to mean that someone really likes or cares about you, but it is actually more about them than it is about you. I caution the individual with a jealous partner. This is a very difficult situation to live in. It gets old fast and fails to grow into a loving, productive relationship most of the time. It comes down to a lack of trust, and if there is no trust there is no foundation for a lasting relationship.

Jealousy is of a lower vibration. Jealousy is a dangerous emotion of an insecure being. If you are with a partner who exhibits this emotion frequently, I recommend you get counseling. Does anything positive come from being jealous? Isn't it just a form of distrust? If you live with those you cannot trust, get out. A relationship is destined for doom if there is a lack of trust.

Are you the jealous type? Why? What are you afraid of? This is such a waste of time and energy. Do you think it makes your partner feel good? Does it make you feel good? If you are comparing a previous relationship to a current one, you are living in the past and that is your issue to resolve, not your partner's.

So many marriages end in battle. Why can't we take what we had, learn from it, and move on? People who cannot let go of feelings of hate, resentment and guilt are prime candidates for illness in the not too distant future. Let it go. Forgive and move on. You'll be a better person for it. The only one you're hurting is yourself. The past is the past and there is no point in dwelling in it. Take the lessons from the experience and move on. Life on earth is short, priceless, and full of opportunity.

If we polled the masses, we could come up with an astounding and colorful array of relationship varieties. For those who are not happy, where do you muster the energy to get through your day? Are you doing it for the kids? I sure hope not. Ultimately the only message you send to your children is that living an unhappy life is how they themselves should tolerate living. If you accept it, why shouldn't they? This is NOT what you want for your children, right? You'd be the first to want them in a happy, fulfilling relationship. But the funny thing about kids is that they learn from their parents. They will learn to love, laugh, and stick up for themselves if you do. If you do not, they will lack self-esteem and the same communications skills that you do. If there is abuse in the household, they will most likely be an abuser or a victim in their own adult relationships. Verbal abuse is often just as harmful as physical abuse. Your children will learn from you. 'Do as I say, not as I do', just doesn't work.

Every once in a while, you will meet the two divorced individuals that end up as great friends. These are the individuals who should be giving marriage/ divorce classes or counseling. It is that these individuals see beyond the letdown and learn from their past experience.

Life is a giant classroom. Learn from what works, and learn from what doesn't. It is the individual that does not grow through or get out of what isn't working that is in trouble, or as I would say, they are emotionally constipated in their relationship.

Some of us are very fortunate in our relationship choices and some of us are not so fortunate. Maybe you ended up in that not-so-great relationship, only to have that spectacular child or children. I'd say that was a success, not a failure. But remember, it is your interpretation that matters most. An individual with a low self-esteem would see this as a failed relationship or that they are a failure. Someone with an intact self-esteem may have wished for better, but something about this situation must have been meant to be.

Attracting the Wrong Partner

So many individuals spend enormous amounts of time

finding the partner that will make them happy. Where are they going with this? For one, if an individual cannot find happiness from within, they are not likely to attract a partner that will do it for them. Yes, maybe temporarily it will appear that they have found happiness, but it will usually be short-lived.

Are you attracted to people who are needy, depressed, emotionally unstable, or never seem to be happy? If you exhibit these qualities, do you expect others to be attracted to you? Most would not find themselves drawn to these characteristics, so don't be this person.

Once you are able to find what makes you happy as an individual, you are much more likely to find a partner to share and participate in your happiness. People generally attract what they project outwardly.

No one is going to come in and fix you if you cannot do it yourself. You may attract a partner who likes to be in control, but not likely to attract a partner who you can evolve with.

Find what you love. Whether it is a hobby, a job or volunteer work, once you become passionate about life and happy in what you do, you will be a magnet for a more fulfilling relationship.

Blood-Sucking Relatives

For many individuals, family gatherings can be a source of stress, especially around holidays and other events. Expectations are that all will go just right, and when it doesn't, the shit will typically hit the fan and feelings will be hurt. It is so sad that relief will come after the event is over, but the damage is done and preconceptions and dread about next year have already begun. Does any of this sound familiar to you? I hope not, but unfortunately I can see and feel the stress pour off of people, especially as the holidays approach.

This is a difficult situation to remedy. Relatives are difficult to avoid especially during the holidays. There is no easy solution for this, but my best recommendation is to make it your goal to keep it light.

Someone gave me excellent advice long ago. I use it to this day and it works every single time. If you find yourself in a heated or potentially volatile confrontation, don't engage. Do not react or give the instigator the benefit of your wit, anger, or retaliation. This will only fuel the fire. The most difficult component is to avoid engaging, but once you do this, you will see how well it works—every time. Use this in any argumentative circumstance and you will always be better for it.

Friend or Parasite?

Do you have any friends who suck your emotions dry? Do they call everyday just to complain about something? Do they do everything better than you, or constantly remind you that you are not doing something right? Do they spend an hour on the phone complaining about the same thing they complained about last year? Can you get a word in edgewise? These individuals have more parasitic qualities than good friend qualities. Rid yourself of parasites! Whether they are in your intestines or in your social circles, they serve no benefit.

Slowly make yourself less and less available. Eventually they will find another host to latch on to, supporting their toxicity. Just don't let it be you. You will be surprised the hours that will free up in your day. This will ultimately open up the door for beneficial friendships, allow romantic relationships to blossom, or even new ones to evolve.

You may feel sorry for this individual as you let them go from your life. You may even have to endure some anger or sadness from this individual, which may leave you feeling guilty. When you do, remember this; a true friend will be there for you, and they nourish your soul just as you nourish theirs. You could go months and sometimes even years, but a good friend remains a good friend. No strings attached.

Chapter 9

Emotionally CONSTIPATED

From a psychological perspective, constipated people can be regarded as misers. They are trying to hold onto things, including their own waste. A type of hoarder, you may say. What does this have to do with constipation? Everything!

Did you ever clean out an attic, basement or even just a closet? How did you feel after you were finished? Did you feel a bit lighter, more energetic and less cluttered? Most would agree that it feels fabulous.

I encourage my constipated patients to get rid of an object that they have not used in the past five years, so they can begin to think in terms of 'letting go'. Surprisingly, this often results in the bowels moving again.

Your JUDGEMENTAL Ways

The famous author Paulo Coelho once wrote, "We can never judge the lives of others, because each person knows only their own pain and renunciation. It's one thing to feel that you are on the right path, but it's another to think that yours is the only path."

In my opinion, being judgmental is one of the most common forms of emotional constipation. It serves little purpose to you or those you judge. Most people find themselves judging others as a way of making themselves feel superior, but sadly, this is not usually the case. The reality is that those who judge the most are typically insecure and are just grasping for reasons to feel better about themselves.

What makes people lack empathy and appear so cold? Besides insecurity, there are some mental disorders that may be to blame. Steve Jobs was thought to have Narcissistic Personality Disorder. Anyone who knew him would agree, yet he served a great purpose during his short life on earth. He lacked empathy for many, and was well known for his arrogance and self-centered ways.

Those suffering from Obsessive-Compulsive Personality Disorder will find fault in almost anyone. They typically say or think that those in their surrounding are too fat or thin, that they are not clean enough, or they dress or look horrible. They can criticize almost every aspect of a person. This is a very unfortunate scenario and is very difficult to overcome. These individuals are very difficult to be around. If you ask them, it is never their intention to hurt or offend anyone.

These are just a few examples of actual disorders that explain the harshness. They know no other way and rarely will be cured of their judgmental ways. You may have a few of these people in your life, but at least now, you yourself may be able look at them with a bit more empathy. Try as hard as you can to find the sympathy and not judge them too harshly.

On a milder note, most of us judge all the time. We may not say anything, but we think it. We do not wish harm on anyone, but we judge people based on what we think is right or wrong. When did "we" become such experts?

I, myself, found that I was doing this more frequently at the grocery store than I'd like to admit. I found myself watching 50 year-old people walking as if they were 80 years old. Looking in their grocery cart, I thought I knew why. I hated when I did this. It did not make me feel good about myself and it served the target of my judgment no purpose.

If you want to experience the lighter, happier life of the non-judgmental person, I recommend the following. Putting this simple tool in place will change your life for the better and for those who believe in karma, you'll have a lot to look forward to.

The next time you find yourself negatively judging someone, turn it to the opposite. If, for example, you judge someone who is overweight, send them wishes of health and happiness. Now, when I find myself in the grocery store, I do the same. This takes the responsibility off me (not that it was any of my business anyway) and leaves them with some healing wishes that they will absolutely benefit from—whether I know them or not.

Apply this to any situation you tend to judge. In a way, you will be paying it forward, and the good wishes you sent out will leave you feeling refreshed and positive. It will become one of the little things that make your day so much better.

This is my favorite quote that hangs in my office:

> *A person who blames others has not begun his/her education. A person who blames him/herself has begun his/her education. A person who blames no one has finished his/her education. The goal is no judgment. Nothing good, nothing bad.*
>
> —anonymous.

ANXIETY: An Unfortunate Dilemma

Nearly 7-million individuals suffer from anxiety, and sometimes to extremes that are sadly out of proportion to what the actual event or situation is. Many sit and anticipate disaster, or worry incessantly about family, work, health or money. The physical and emotional toll can be crippling.

Symptoms can range from mild, such as feeling tense; to severe, and actually having symptoms similar to a heart attack. Many suffer from ulcers, diarrhea and/or constipation as a result. Anxiety can and will take a physical toll on the body. The potential for creativity and pleasurable life experiences will be stunted in those that suffer from chronic anxiety.

Once medical conditions such as hyperthyroidism, adrenal fatigue and hormone imbalance are ruled out or remedied, one can begin to seek out what may help overcome anxiety. In my practice, women from puberty through menopause that suffer from unexplainable anxiety often test very deficient in progesterone. Blood levels are often normal, but saliva testing reveals low levels especially when compared to estrogen.

Evaluating hormone levels via blood work fails to look at the ratio between estrogen and progesterone, a big miss when it comes to helping women with anxiety and insomnia. Men often suffer from anxiety if testosterone levels are low.

Someone suffering from adrenal fatigue is described as the person that feels that if someone were to give him or her just one more thing to do, they would crumble. The inability to cope with things that are not life threatening may be a sign of adrenal fatigue. I know all too well, as I have had to address adrenal fatigue personally. Thankfully, supplementation works well.

Medications do not fix the problem or even begin to uncover what the problem may be, but many individuals will gladly take the medication that will at least provide a comforting blanket for what ails them. What they do not realize is that most of these medications cause dependency. They will most likely develop a tolerance for them that may result in increasing the dosage or switching to other medications.

Activities that reduce anxiety include exercise, meditation, yoga, Qigong and prayer. Supplements that support adrenal function (adaptogens) are often helpful, but don't ignore the basics. Omega-3 fatty acids (fish oils), magnesium and B vitamins all play an important role in emotional health.

Other alternatives that have been successful include hypnosis, acupuncture and Reiki. EFT (Emotional Freedom Technique) has shown tremendous promise with individuals suffering from anxiety and a host of other illnesses. There is plenty of free information available to you via the Internet— www.EFTuniverse.com would be a great place to start.

What is actually worthy of the impact that anxiety has on you? Why do you torture yourself? You may want to ask yourself whether the emotions you are feeling will be as important or vivid in a year, a week, or even an hour. You cannot distance yourself from what life may have in store for you, but you can relinquish your attempts to control situations and find yourself pleasantly basking in an "it is what it is" attitude. There is a priceless "peace" of mind that comes with this way of thinking. Enjoyment and gratitude of what life has to offer becomes the focus, rather than the crippling thoughts of what may go wrong.

The next time you find yourself caught in those negative thought patterns that induce anxiety, imagine the best possible results rather than the worst-case scenario. Loved ones arriving home safe, problems at work being solved with ease, medical test results coming back clear, and so forth. The more you put this new way of thinking into practice, the more automatic it becomes. Sometimes just the shift from resistance to acceptance is all that is needed to easy anxiety, allowing us to be open to all experiences and good to come.

Anger

I'm not sure if I agree with the popular saying, "Holding on to anger is like holding a hot coal, you are the only one who gets burned". Angry people can change the atmosphere of a room without even saying a word. Because we are very intuitive, anger is easily palpable and the discomfort of being around an angry person can easily have a negative physical impact on the body. Most experience this in the gut, neck and shoulders as stress and tension. If you are frequently in contact with an angry person, you feel almost weightless when they leave the house, workplace or wherever you spend time with them. Even the air becomes easier to breathe.

Why do some people seem to get angry at the drop of a hat? It is most likely the result of a parent who was frequently angry, and becomes a learned behavior for many. Chemical imbalances, medication side effects, constipation, unstable blood sugars, insecurity, and a feeling of loss of control are also common causes of angry outbursts.

Anger is a powerful emotion that can take a toll on physical health as well as the emotional health of those surrounded by it. Anger can be loud, with vulgar language; or it can be seething, like a volcano ready to blow.

Long-term effects of anger are anxiety, high blood pressure, headaches and digestive issues. I feel that cancer is more easily manifested in chronically angry people.

I doubt that you will get any angry person to admit they enjoy feeling this way, but most feel helpless as they lack the tools to diffuse the outbursts that disrupt the lives of so many. The most important thing to remember is that your anger outburst will almost never fix the situation. It almost always makes things worse.

The next time you feel yourself building up steam, ready for an eruption, take a deep breath and wait 30 seconds. This seems like an eternity in the heat of the situation, but it may be all you need to prevent the outburst.

Aerobic exercise is a great outlet for those who suffer from frequent episodes of rage. It also benefits your physical health, which is the exact opposite of what suppressed anger will do. If your anger is choked down quietly, you must be careful of the potential physical ailments that can easily manifest. Blood pressure elevations and aneurysms are two examples of what swallowed anger can do.

There are many online helpful resources on the topic of anger and different tools that may help. Anger is only one letter short of danger, and many people are hurt in its path.

As far as supplementation, homeopathic remedies may be one of the more effective supplements available. Homeopathic remedies do not interfere with medications, making them safe for everyone. Because there are many personality types, one remedy does not fit all. Someone with education and experience in homeopathy would be able to point you in the right direction. Nux vomica and lycopodium are a few of the remedies used in the treatment of anger. Combination remedies are also available.

"Anger is never without a reason, but seldom with a good one."
—Benjamin Franklin

Fear

Too many people live in a constant state of fear; fear for themselves, fear for their children; fear of the unknown, and on and on. Fear is like a tight leash that allows you to go nowhere. I love the acronym: **F**alse **E**xpectations **A**ssumed **R**eal. Fear is not protective; it is controlling and harmful. Placing your fears on others is even worse than just having your own. What good does being fearful bring? NONE. It does not save you from danger, as there is no danger. The fear you have is an illusion that you have created in your mind. All illusions have the power to seem very real.

Please do not confuse fear for intuition or a sixth sense warning. Intuition is something that I have tried to help my children develop. Again, I am not telling them what to believe, but rather what to pay attention to. When you develop the ability to trust your intuition, there is no reason to be afraid.

Guilt

Typically, guilt is described as a feeling of responsibility or remorse for some offense, crime, wrongdoing, etc.—whether real or imagined. Unfortunately, our own moral beliefs may set us up to be extremely judgmental of ourselves, therefore constipating our potential in life.

Guilt becomes problematic when one feels responsible for a situation that they had no control over. This self-punishing behavior tends to be a repetitive theme for the individual. He or she cannot be the actual victim, so they take on the guilt, which is a victim-like attitude all in itself.

Individuals that feel guilty in situations that they had no control over, typically suffer from feelings of worthlessness and inferiority.

People pleasers that often try to make everyone happy, often feel guilty when they cannot. Why is everybody else's destiny and happiness your responsibility in the first place? This is a very enabling behavior that benefits no one and usually leads to feelings of resentment.

Religious guilt is a common situation that has many well-intending people feeling as if they are "bad" in the eyes of God or their cultural ways. Missing church on Sunday, not donating to the church, or marrying outside of their religious denomination or culture is just some of the reasons people feel guilt. I have nothing against any religion, as it brings structure and comfort to so many; but many individuals are carrying unnecessary guilt, which can negatively impact one's psyche.

People who often suffer feelings of guilt are sabotaging and crippling their potential. These individuals commonly feel inferior, lack self-esteem and self-worth, and will likely prevent future success in their life. Guilt is extremely self-destructive and rarely worth the time and energy devoted to it.

Letting go of guilt and learning to forgive ourselves for being human is a major step in moving forward in life. It is well worth the effort, even if it means questioning your religious or cultural beliefs.

If you have truly wronged someone, and it nags at you, ask for forgiveness. Even if the object of your request denies your forgiveness or is not living anymore, the benefits of just asking for that forgiveness have an amazing impact. You are much more likely to let the guilt go.

Attracting the Negative

The Law of Attraction, especially to the negative, is demonstrated so easily in today's society. The Universe does not decipher the fact that you may like or dislike the subject, but will draw to it. So if we want to rid the world of war, stop focusing on the war and start focusing on peace. Stop drawing your attention to bad politicians, focus on the good ones instead, and so on.

The Law of Attraction brings in the good as well as the bad. It is your every thought. There are hundreds of excellent books that can help you fine-tune your skill of using the Law of Attraction to draw in the good.

Just as easy as it is to attract the good, you can just as easily attract the negative. My own example involves deer. Although I have nothing against them, I have developed a fear of hitting them as a result of my first accident.

It was before six in the morning and I was on my way to work at the hospital. It was late November, and although there was no snow on the ground, it was a cold dark morning. I frequently use my high beams, as the parkway is dark and not well lit. Deer are a common sighting, but I really never gave it too much thought until I slammed into one doing about 55-60mph. Needless to say, giant Bambi did not survive. My car did not survive either. Lucky not to be hurt, life went on.

Although I am not typically the fearing type, I began to develop a fear of hitting more deer. "What are the odds of hitting another deer?" I would tell myself all the time, as I just could not stop worrying about it. I truly believe that being fearful and thinking about it all the time was part of the reason that I hit two more deer over the next few years. How could I break this pattern of negative thinking and reduce my fear that ultimately became a negative attraction?

Because the topic would come up often and I happen to be surrounded by some very amazing and gifted people, I had the opportunity to receive the best advice that continues to work (you cannot see me right now as I am looking for wood to knock on) many years later. I was told to put a protective force field around my car, imaginative of course, for a safe drive. As silly as this sounds, it is working and I am not thinking about hitting deer anymore.

Don't focus on what you are lacking in your life, because all you will attract is more "lack of". Focus on what you have and are grateful for, and more of that is sure to come your way. Focus on peace rather than war. Focus on what's great about this country, not about what is in a state of despair. Focus on the positive stories and acts of kindness in the world rather than the sad and unspeakable. Do this to everything in your immediate surrounding. This small switch of thinking will bring a tremendous amount of peace and happiness to your life.

Emotional Affects Physical

I recently had a woman come in who had just been diagnosed with recurrent breast cancer, only this time they had found that it spread to her liver. They told her it was a "small" area. She relayed to me that she had a sister who was diagnosed with cancer five years back and had beaten it. Her sister made some huge lifestyle changes and continues to practice them today. When I questioned her on why she didn't do what her sister did, she stated that she "didn't believe in all that stuff," and besides, her sister was "no expert". She admits that may not have been in her best interest, as her sister remains cancer-free today. My heart ached for her. It is very funny how people will not take good advice from those they are closest to.

Her history revealed that her past 20 years had been stressful. I knew in my heart that this was partly the reason that the cancer had returned, so I asked her the following difficult question, "What are you going to change about your stressful life that would give your body good reason to live?" A bad marriage or relationship should not be tolerated. If you were the body of an individual that lived a stressful, unhappy life, would you want to stay or check out? Me personally—I'd want out. I knew that if her body had nothing to recover for, it wouldn't.

Your surroundings play a huge role on your emotional and physical health. Surrounding yourself with positive people who bring in peace, love and humor is better than any medication. The sick individual has a far greater chance of a rapid recovery in this environment. On the contrary, an environment that is stressful and unhappy is unlikely to facilitate success when it comes to healing.

Whether you are a patient, family member, healthcare provider or friend, please do not take the surrounding environment lightly. Healing can and will be inhibited if the surroundings are not positive and peaceful. I wish hospitals would heed this information.

SUMMARY

Constipated emotions constipate our lives, preventing us from many potentially rewarding experiences. If you feel that you relate to any of the above situations, congratulations! You have accomplished the very important step of recognition, and can now move forward in freeing yourself from the sluggishness that these emotions can cause.

Individuals who are not emotionally constipated are

calming and soothing to be around. They will never drag you down and will almost always lift you up. They rarely get sucked into drama, which enables them to think clearly and not judge the situation. Emotional endurance comes naturally, which adds years to a person's life.

Chapter 10

CONSTIPATION in Birth, Death & Spirituality

My life as a midwife has exposed me to what many may describe as the most beautiful moment of life. Birth. Nine months of anticipation, waiting for that incredible moment.

There is however, constipation in childbirth. I am not speaking of the literal complication of a backed up bowel that is common among pregnant women, but rather the attempt to control the whole experience of childbirth.

From the moment the desired pregnancy is confirmed, the expectant mother envisions her delivery. I will speak specifically of first-time moms and their typical scenario of expectations as the imminent birth approaches. Now let me remind you that I have over 25 years of experience on the labor wing; so to avoid becoming constipated in the art of childbirth, listen up.

Many first-time mothers know how they want to deliver—natural. They want to do it without the help of pain medication or epidural anesthesia. I would venture to say with accuracy that maybe only 10-15 percent will actually do this, although I will give them credit and support the birth anyway they want to do it. Actually, that is the definition of a midwife. Midwife means "with woman", no matter what her desires for birth are.

I am personally a fan of epidural anesthesia. I don't sound like much of a midwife do I? A good epidural will help facilitate the most beautiful birth. Because the delivery is a bit more controlled there is often very little to repair, as we can let the birth of the head deliver very slow and gradual. Because episiotomies are becoming a thing of the past, there are very few complications as a result of extensive tearing. For those of you who are unfamiliar as to what an episiotomy is, it is a cut made to better facilitate the baby's head as it delivers from the vagina. The problem is that it often extends, possibly even into the rectum.

Back to why I like epidurals. When you watch women giving birth without the help of an epidural, the exhaustion that often takes place takes them somewhere else. Between the pain and exhaustion, I feel that she has "checked out". This is a protective modality in childbirth, and also what I feel is responsible for the infamous amnesia.

Women with epidurals are more of a participant in the birth of their children. They still experience the urge to push (most of the time) that guides them through the process. They are typically less exhausted and therefore have better bonding experiences with their babies afterward.

In 25 years, I have yet to see the woman paralyzed by an epidural. Many mothers come in afraid of receiving an epidural because they heard of someone having horrible complications. This stuns me, as I have heard it over and over from new and expecting moms; yet in over 25 years, I have yet to see it. What would possess anyone to tell a pregnant woman anything but a nice story? Every pregnant woman seems to be a magnet for someone's horror story, which is usually fabricated to some extent. This scares people and then they spend a good part of the pregnancy dreading something that is not likely to happen. This is part of what sets the stage for constipation in childbirth.

The Birth Plan

The birth plan is a set of desires that the expectant mother and father would like to incorporate into the birth experience. For the most part, they are within reason and include the desire to be able walk during labor, be off the monitor at times, for dad to be able to cut the cord, etc. But for some, the control is much tighter than that. They request no IV, we are not to offer pain medications ever, no talking during the birth, and I have even had requests for no cesarean section under any circumstances.

I have learned to read these and keep my comments and thoughts to myself. The more demanding the birth plan, the more likely this mom will be disappointed, as this is one venue she will not have that much control over. This is typically not an issue for the under 30 crowd, as they are more likely to be go-with-the-flow. The younger the mother, the less expectations they have with the experience, and the more go-with-the-flow they are. I am not trying to stereotype, but the woman who waits until she has the perfect husband, the perfect job, the perfect house, and the perfect amount of money in her bank account before having the baby is usually the controlling type that generally has a harder time in labor. What people fail to realize is that we (the staff) do not have much control over how your labor will go, and it humors us that you think you do. Ask ANY labor nurse; the more expectations and requests you have on a birth plan, the higher the chances are for a cesarean section. Don't ask me why, but this is always the case. I think it may have something to do with the universe reminding you that you are not in total control and there needs to be a part of you that is flexible. The very structured birth plan makes the staff feel as if you think they are incompetent and wouldn't do what's best for you without these guidelines. This does not tend to start the relationship off very well.

Those who come in and say, "I'd like to do it this way but I am open to change," are the people who tend to have the best experience. They may have even had a complicated delivery, but because their baby is born and safe, the experience as a whole was positive.

In the case where the structured birth plan was not followed accordingly, the outcome may be perfect, but this is not how the parents will perceive it. This is where the perception of childbirth becomes constipated.

Birth seems to be the best experience when it happens on its own terms. The mother with an open mind who can trust her body will usually get through the pregnancy with a graceful strength that leaves everyone in awe.

Death

In general, birth is a beautiful experience, the beginning

of all possibilities, and what seems to be for an infinite amount of time.

But from that instant of birth, comes the absolute guarantee of death. As terrible as it sounds, it is inevitable and yet we fight it so. We surround it with drama and sadness. Now you are thinking, "obviously this author is cold-hearted, unfeeling and lacks sensitivity." No I am not, and yes, the death of a loved one would impact me as much as you, the reader. But I have to wonder, isn't there a simpler way to cope with something that is, and always will be, inevitable? I can't say that I have figured things out, but I am trying to approach the inevitability of death with a new wisdom and calmness.

Perhaps there is a new way to think of death; from the eyes of an elder, or from the eyes of an untarnished child diagnosed with an incurable or terminal illness. I am often in awe of terminal cancer patients. Their strength, insight and wisdom melt my heart. I often think that their own death would be easier if they were able to share their wisdom and insight with those around them. Instead, many hold all that good wisdom to themselves, as death is perceived taboo and is not a topic that is freely discussed between family members. Denial at it's finest.

Have you ever experienced the death of a loved one, a patient, or other experience? Most would hardly call it a bad experience. It is almost always described as surreal, peaceful and beautiful. Ask any hospice nurse what he or she thinks about the emotions and experiences that surround death. You may be surprised. Hospice employees are anything but depressed, anxiety ridden or unhappy; that is a thought to ponder.

I had the unfortunate experience of being with a 17-year-old boy seconds after a car accident that took his young life. How could that be beautiful and peaceful, you ask? I am a firm believer that when it is your time, it is your time. I know this boy had no pain, and he did not experience the time to be scared. In an instant he was taken, and for him, the transit was immediate, painless and peaceful. For those of us at the scene, which included my husband and children, peaceful was not our initial reaction. But these thoughts were what provided all of us with comfort once the shock of what we had witnessed had worn off.

I stayed with this boy feeling helpless, and only able to say over and over, "It's OK to go". Knowing there was nothing anyone could do to save this boy, it was all I could think to do. I did not want to walk away from that car because I didn't want to admit to my children or husband that this boy was gone and there was nothing more that could be done, except to wait for first responders.

I asked for and did receive a beautiful sign awhile later that all was well and he transitioned easily. A very brilliant golden light in the back of my head (out of my physical visual field) told me all was well. How did I interpret that? I just asked for a sign that he was OK. Ask and you shall receive. Because I am a human and my "left brain" gets in the way, I admit I always try to rationalize what I get, then kick myself for not saying thank you for my obvious answer. His parents did find comfort in knowing he had not suffered.

I was once close with a Catholic priest dying of terminal cancer. Father Bob and I met shortly after he was diagnosed. I was a fairly new, very young labor and delivery nurse. He was the hospital Chaplin and his room was on the same floor I worked. It all started by asking him to join us for dinner, then eventually bringing him dinner, and eventually medicating his pain from bone cancer. In hindsight, I wish I had taped some of our conversations, as death was a fascinating conversation because we both knew it was inevitable at some point and did not feel the need to protect each other from that fact.

I did ask Father Bob to give me a sign that all is well from the other side, but made him promise that he wouldn't scare me. I still hear his loud laughter to this day at my very serious request. Well, that message did come loud and clear one evening as I left work. It had been a week or so since he had passed. I looked up at the window, where he used to wave goodbye, and saw the most amazing golden cross. It was blinding, but very real! Of course my human "left brain" could not accept my sign and continued to feel the need to explain what I saw. My "left brain" was sure it must have been a reflection from somewhere, my "right brain" held no doubts of the origin of the cross. Thanks Father Bob, you will never be forgotten.

How odd that someone who has spent most of her working life with birth now finds herself comforting the thoughts of death and what is beyond. Many years ago, during an Intuitive Healing class, I admitted being very drawn to the idea of helping others transition at the time of death. I wanted to be that person (in spirit) that would tell you of the beauty on the other side. You would hear a voice and find comfort and peace there as you yourself left the human side of life. I wanted to be the first to introduce you to your loved ones including your past pets. I was sure this is how it goes and wanted to be part of it. My intuitive instructor then said, "What makes you think your work needs to be done from that side?" So here I sit today wondering if this is part of the work I am to do on "this side". I'm not sure how to make people more comfortable with the reality of death, but I am trying.

Religious & Spiritual Constipation

Talk about hot topics. I have only recently become comfortable in my own skin when it comes to religion. Being raised Roman Catholic was not a bad experience, but it never quite resonated with me. I felt a failure to my children that I did not establish a good religious foundation. How would they survive as adults if I failed to provide a rock solid foundation?

I'm over the guilt now, as it only provides a breeding ground for illness and insecurity. I envy people who find comfort in their religion, for no matter what the religion, it is the right one for them. I believe all religions lead to the same universal creator, known as God.

God is all-loving, all-forgiving, and supports us no matter what path we are on. I also believe He/ She has a great sense of humor. We are all here on this plane of our own accord and to fulfill a specific life purpose. We have been here before and we will be here again. I do not believe in hell, but do believe we can create one here on earth. I believe all is as it should be...all the time. God is all-perfect.

Unfortunately many believe that it should be their way or it is wrong. This thinking has torn families apart, that otherwise may have gotten along just fine. Wars have been started and populations have been destroyed based on religious beliefs. The God that I am familiar with would not pit one religion against another.

If we would all just focus on being helpful, kind

and nonjudgmental in our immediate surroundings, we would all be in a better place. A "pay it forward" type attitude serves everyone, and it does not have to be in the form of money. This is the best religion.

If you are like me and do not feel connected to a specific religion, please do not feel lost. Being well connected to God, the Spirit or the Universe does not have to be defined by any specific religion. It is the good you do, the life you live, and your ultimate essence that will give you roots to grow spiritually and radiate infectiously to your family and surrounding contacts.

Chapter 11

YOU, NOT CONSTIPATED!

Your Personal Power

Have you ever had the day that everything went right? You don't know where your energy came from, and you can't find the plug that you must be attached to in order to feel this "charged". You couldn't be pessimistic if you tried, and the world just can't penetrate this great feeling no matter what is going on. This feeling comes when you are in what is commonly referred to as your "personal power". I refer to it as "unconstipated". When you are in this state, you are actually tapped into a higher realm and your ability to create and manifest are in their prime. This is the state you strive to be in!

Unfortunately, most of us only get a glimmer of ourselves in our personal power from time to time. Imagine what would occur if we were in this state most of the time. What would you do? (Let me remind you that when you are in this state, you are already doing what you love). Who would be the people you surround yourself

with? Who would you remove from your surroundings?
Be honest, and I don't care how related they are to you.
When you are in this space, you glow. You absolutely
radiate. People can feel you. You are infectious and
those around you want what you've got.

Instead of wasting your time trying to be the martyr
for everyone else, be the person working in his or her
highest power. This will create the biggest positive
change with a trickle-down effect to all who know you.
There is no better way to teach than by setting a good
example. Too many people, especially women, spend
most of their life trying to be the perfect parent, the
perfect spouse, or the best friend who always comes to the
rescue. Not that this is bad, but if taken to an extreme, it
sets up a horrible midlife reality that screams of personal
deprivation. Be good to yourself, now and always. Do
not give up all that you love for the sake of your family.
This is a poor example to set for your children and a
surefire way to enable your spouse. An enabled spouse is
a tremendous amount of work.

Be passionate about many different things,
continue to learn, set goals and go places. No one can
make you happy if you can't do it yourself.

The Law of Attraction

One of the most basic universal truths is the Law of
Attraction. Simply put, what you think of you will attract.
I will recommend you read *The Secret* or *As a Man
Thinkith,* as they will help to redirect your thoughts in a
positive, abundant way.

I have always dreamed of a house on the water.
Born under the Cancer sign, I am a magnet to the water

and can't imagine my life without water in my sight. At the time, we had two young children. My husband was an undercover detective and I was a part-time labor and delivery nurse who was back in school for midwifery. Financially, things were tight but we were hanging in there. Every once in a while we would drive along the waterfront of the Niagara region and look at the houses that had the waterfront that I hoped and wished to someday own.

Then one day, the ball began to roll. I have to say, this is an absolute example of what we have the power to manifest in our lives. We were driving to a relative's house to meet on the day my husband's grandmother passed away. Lewiston and Youngstown, NY are beautiful small towns that happen to be situated along the lower Niagara River about 5-10 miles from the base of Niagara Falls. The view across the river faces west to Canada and it boasts some of the best sunsets I have seen anywhere in the world. As we were driving, there was a house for sale that the sun was setting on, making the stained glass windows absolutely glow. It was on the waterside of the street. I specifically remember hitting my husband's arm, laughing as I said, "Imagine living in that house!" I'm not sure what happened in that moment, but something did. I became obsessed!

Online, the house was listed for well over what we could ever afford. Many people would have stopped right there, but not me; and I'm not sure why. I took a drive myself down to that house on the river. It had been empty for a bit, so I pulled my car down deep into the driveway so it was hidden from the street. I got out and walked to the back of the house.

The back porch was a huge covered area with the

most amazing view I had ever seen. I cupped my hand and peeked into the windows of this amazing house that I was growing very attached to. Small kitchen—I could live with that. The family room with a stone fireplace and a big living room on the other side of the kitchen was all I could see from the large windows on the porch. What possessed me to check the door, I don't even know. As I turned the handle and found it open, my heart raced and the adrenalin kicked in. Realizing I was totally breaking the law and trespassing, I went in. I felt as if the house was inviting me. With my heart pounding, I ran up the stairs, through the house, and immediately thought it was move-in ready. I got back out on the porch fairly quick, for fear I'd be caught. I called my husband (remember, he's a cop) and proceeded to be scolded for breaking the law. Needless to say, he made a few phone calls and on the same day was down there looking at this "out of reach" house falling in love with it, right alongside me.

A very long, sweet story made short: Six months later we owned that house for a fraction of what it was listed for. I credit my husband's persistence, my intentions, and the universe that listened with open ears. For a million years, you could rationalize why this could never be possible; but it happened. As I am writing this book, I am sitting on that beautiful porch on a June summer day, still in awe of the beautiful view for which I will never take for granted.

This was not the only experience of manifestation from using the law of attraction for me. The building that my business Journey II Health resides in was acquired, renovated and open for business six months after my husband found it. I was pretty much laughed at by three separate banks, and yet here I am. You can rationalize all day long why any of this should not have worked out. This is what most people do. They feel it is out of reach, and shut the door. This is where most people stop. What a mistake. If you want something, go for it! Don't let your own negative thoughts or negative people in your atmosphere talk you down. By the law of attraction, anything—whether it be health, relationships, material items or success—is within your reach. There are an abundance of books written on the topic. I highly recommend you read them in order to stay focused and motivated in order to get what you want.

Healing

What I love about Journey II Health is that when a client comes in, they have already taken the responsibility to walk through the door. Now I will be the first to tell you that there is a tremendous amount of healing that takes place amongst these walls, and it has little to do with me. Most individuals step through the door with the intention to heal. This is the most important aspect, and they came in with it. I am very upfront in telling them that I will not be the one to heal them, rather they will intuitively find the right combination of therapies, or one single therapy. We will help facilitate the path, but they will do the healing. As simple as this sounds, it works. I make some recommendations to start and then they are off on their own, well-supported all the way.

What heals some does not heal others. We have ignored and suppressed our own intuitive abilities that are vital to our health and well-being. The biggest obstacle is getting the client to tap into this intuition and listen. Too many people do not trust their "gut". I have taught my children from a very early age to trust their gut feelings, as they are correct 90 percent of the time. (Actually, I believe it is 100 percent of the time, but I will allow ten percent for being human). We have a variety of clients who come through our doors. They range from just wanting some form of detoxification, to the terminally ill.

By the time a person who is terminally ill comes to see me, he or she has already gone through all the well-known stages of grieving. Although Elisabeth Kubler-Ross is well known for her *Five Stages of Grief,* I believe there should be six; with "shock" being placed at number one on the list. Whether it is diagnosis of illness, an accident, or the loss of a loved one, I believe that shock comes first. This is not such a bad thing, as it may play a protective role in buffering the true impact of the given situation. The well-known stages of grief include denial, anger, bargaining, depression and acceptance. When my patients get to me, most have worked through the emotional stages and have come to accept what life has dealt them. This enables the client to begin the healing process. "Healing" does not always mean, "curing". People who heal can still die. This sounds like a conflict, but actually it is quite beautiful.

Remember, from the moment you were born, you were guaranteed, at some point, to die. Imagine being allowed to do so without fear. If you have not read the works of Bernie Seigel, I highly recommend them on this subject. He has a beautiful and eloquent way of describing the healing process. I highly recommend his book, *Love, Medicine and Miracles.*

I had the beautiful experience of working with a woman who became a close friend. She gave death a run for its money and outlived a terminal diagnosis by at least seven years. Her name was Kim and she was the strongest woman I have ever met. Kim had been given a terminal diagnosis of stage-four breast cancer and she was not going down without a fight. She had been battling her cancer for nine years before it finally took her life. If you met this woman, you would find it hard to believe she was sick.

When I met her, the only sign of illness would have been the new hair growth—which actually looked quite stylish—from her last round of chemotherapy. She had decided that she would not continue the chemo, as it just made her feel bad. She did see an iridologist who had placed her on a strict nutritional program. Kim came to Journey II Health to see if there was anything else she could do. She had family vacations to plan and even a few trips to St. John's, one of which I was fortunate enough to experience with her. We needed to maintain the vibrancy and keep her strong.

As with all my cancer patients, I always ask what happened in the years before the cancer diagnosis. Most often I get an answer easily. A stressful marker or event in one's life will usually trigger an illness. In Kim's case it was her daughter's open-heart surgeries years before. I am not saying that it was the event that caused the cancer, but more the emotions created by the event and how Kim processed them—or didn't.

Misdiagnoses lead to more than one open-heart surgery for her young daughter. In the end, after more than one surgery and a month on life support, her daughter recovered and even went on to becoming a champion high school swimmer. The anger toward the physicians in error was palpable, even many years later. This, I believe, is what fueled the cancer. She just couldn't let go of the anger. Kim out-lived her diagnosis by seven years. It was a life of quality and she and her family traveled frequently. She remained the captain of her own ship right up until the end. Being an equal player in your healing process is the key. She lived a better life for it.

I have seen and heard many stories of remarkable healing or miracles. I truly believe with every fiber of my being that the individual facilitates the process 90 percent, and that we as outsiders only play a very small part. Yes, I do believe in God and the power of prayer.

Intuition & Health

YOU ARE THE BEST DOCTOR YOU WILL EVER HAVE. Doctors, specialists, naturopaths and other healers should be viewed as tools that help you gather the information necessary to help YOU make the best choices when it comes to your health and well-being. Unfortunately, many of us become dependent on someone else to "fix" us, as we plead ignorant and don't want to take on the responsibility. Well I am here to remind you that even though your doctor is well-intending and does want to help you; you have to care more, and be willing to take ownership and responsibility when it comes to your health. If not, you will be very disappointed in the outcome.

I love intuition. It is exceptionally accurate and cuts to the chase quicker than any lab test ever could. Unfortunately, medicine today is dictated by the insurance companies and not by the experience or intuitive gifts of the patient or physician. Every medication, lab test, MRI and surgery has to follow a specific sequence in order to be approved. Physicians in this country are practicing more as robots than they are as independent and intelligent thinkers. This may not always be in the patient's best interest.

It always amazes me when people "know" something isn't right. It may be something as serious as cancer or more commonly, something much less serious. They can usually pinpoint right down to organ system or organ. Sadly, many health care providers are not well-versed in the art of listening. It would save an incredible amount of time and money if we would just listen.

There has been very little research done in regards to healthcare professionals using their intuition. Most academics would not be open to discussing or researching a sixth sense. It would be hard to measure and evaluate, and falls into a right brain category in a world of left brain thinkers.

Nurses have been studied to some degree when it comes to intuition. The common conclusion was: the more experience the nurse had, the more accurate her "gut" feeling was. There have been many events in my life as a practicing nurse or midwife that have been intuitively guided. I am thankful that I was open to listening, and I'm sure the patients were too.

Years ago as a young labor and delivery nurse, I had such an experience. Had I not been so persistent to a physician that was not listening, we may have lost that baby and even the mother. I'll call the mother Kelly (not that I remember her name, anyway). Kelly was in active labor and had just received an epidural for pain. This was her third child. Kelly's first baby was born via Cesarean Section for reasons I cannot recall. She had a successful vaginal birth for baby number two, and was currently in active labor with her third baby. As the epidural began to take her pain away, she sensed something was not right. She described a tearing or stretching sensation. The physician in charge was notified immediately and came into the room. Because her vital signs were stable, as was the baby's heart rate, she left the room reassured all was well. I was not reassured.

Something was not right; I could see it in her face. I proceeded to tell my charge nurse and she had the operating room prepared just in case. Lucky for me she listened.

Within 15 minutes, I had a baby whose heart rate was in the 60's (normal is 120-160) and not coming up. My patient was rushed to the OR for an emergency C-Section. Her previously scarred uterus had opened up and the baby was partially in the abdomen when the surgeons got in there. The baby responded very well to minimal resuscitation, and mom and baby both recovered without complication. I often wondered what would have happened if I just ignored that nagging gut feeling and listened to the physician who said that everything was fine. What if the OR was not set up and ready to go? Would we have been able to resuscitate the baby as easily?

So Now...

You and I have built-in gifts to guide us through whatever life has to offer. An unconstipated individual (emotionally and physically) is able to utilize these gifts and this personal power with greater ease than if he or she were constipated. Life is much easier with far less drama.

I hope to have given you some valuable tools so that you may carry on in an unconstipated fashion. You should begin to feel lighter; the worry lifts, the fog lifts, and the crap in your life leaves you effortlessly. The popular saying, "it is what it is" should become your reality and you should be comfortable there.

The more you incorporate a healthy diet into your life, the more addicted you become to feeling good. You won't tolerate feeling sluggish and will do anything in your power to remain in a constipation-free state.

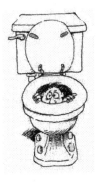

journeyiihealth.com

Notes...

_____

_____

_____

_____

_____

_____

_____

_____

_____

_____

_____

_____

_____

_____

_____

_____

_____

_____

_____

_____

_____

_____

Notes...

Notes...

_____

_____

_____

_____

_____

_____

_____

_____

_____

_____

_____

_____

_____

_____

_____

_____

_____

_____

_____

Notes…

_____

_____

_____

_____

_____

_____

_____

_____

_____

_____

_____

_____

_____

_____

_____

_____

_____

_____

_____

Notes…

YOU, NOT CONSTIPATED!

Notes…

_____

_____

_____

_____

_____

_____

_____

_____

_____

_____

_____

_____

_____

_____

_____

_____

_____

_____

_____

_____

_____

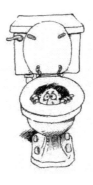

journeyiihealth.com

QUICK ORDER FORM

ONLINE orders:
www.constipatedlife.com OR www.journeyiihealth.com
EMAIL orders:
Joureyiihealth@gmail.com
PHONE orders:
716-298-8603. Have your credit card handy
FAX orders:
716-298-8604. Send this form.
MAIL orders:
Journey II Health, 7311 Porter Rd, Niagara Falls, NY 14304

[ ] **Free Yourself from a CONSTIPATED Life**................... **$16.95**
[ ] **Cape Aloe**.. **$11.50**
[ ] **One Drop Deodorizer**..**$9.50**

Sales Tax: For New York addresses only, please add $8.25% to the book purchase (not supplements).
Shipping: $6.95 for orders less than $50.00. $12.95 for orders less than $100.00. Call for larger orders.

Order Total: _____

Name: _____

Address: _____

City: _____ State: _____

Zip: _____ Telephone: _____

Email: _____
I would like to receive:
[ ] Journey II Health's Monthly Newsletter
[ ] Information on Catherine Stack's Speaking Engagements

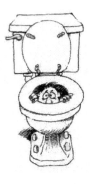

journeyiihealth.com

QUICK ORDER FORM

ONLINE orders:
www.constipatedlife.com OR www.journeyiihealth.com
EMAIL orders:
Joureyiihealth@gmail.com
PHONE orders:
716-298-8603. Have your credit card handy
FAX orders:
716-298-8604. Send this form.
MAIL orders:
Journey II Health, 7311 Porter Rd, Niagara Falls, NY 14304

[   ] **Free Yourself from a CONSTIPATED Life** **$16.95**
[   ] **Cape Aloe** **$11.50**
[   ] **One Drop Deodorizer** **$9.50**

Sales Tax: For New York addresses only, please add $8.25% to the book purchase (not supplements).
Shipping: $6.95 for orders less than $50.00. $12.95 for orders less than $100.00. Call for larger orders.

Order Total: _____

Name: _____

Address: _____

City: _____ State: _____

Zip: _____ Telephone: _____

Email: _____
I would like to receive:
[   ] Journey II Health's Monthly Newsletter
[   ] Information on Catherine Stack's Speaking Engagements

Made in the USA
Lexington, KY
06 March 2015